D0875645

Lifestyle Management in Health and Social Care

Lifestyle Management in Health and Social Care

Edited by

Miranda Thew

Occupational Science and Occupational Therapy Group
Faculty of Health
Leeds Metropolitan University
Leeds

and

Jim McKenna

Professor of Physical Activity and Health
Faculty of Health
Carnegie Research Institute
Leeds Metropolitan University
Leeds

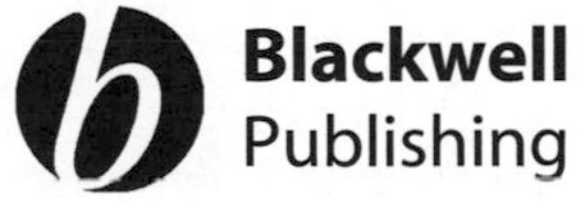

This edition first published 2008

Blackwell Publishing was acquired by John Wiley & Sons in February 2007. Blackwell's publishing programme has been merged with Wiley's global Scientific, Technical, and Medical business to form Wiley-Blackwell.

Registered office
John Wiley & Sons Ltd, The Atrium, Southern Gate, Chichester, West Sussex, PO19 8SQ, United Kingdom

Editorial office
9600 Garsington Road, Oxford, OX4 2DQ, United Kingdom
350 Main Street, Malden, MA 02148-5020, USA

For details of our global editorial offices, for customer services and for information about how to apply for permission to reuse the copyright material in this book please see our website at www.wiley.com/wiley-blackwell.

Library of Congress Cataloging-in-Publication Data

Lifestyle management in health and social care / edited by Miranda Thew.
p. ; cm.
Includes bibliographical references and index.
ISBN-13: 978-1-4051-7114-4 (pbk. : alk. paper)
ISBN-10: 1-4051-7114-6 (pbk. : alk. paper) 1. Lifestyles–Health aspects. 2. Health behavior.
3. Behavior modification. I. Thew, Miranda.
[DNLM: 1. Health Behavior. 2. Counseling–methods. 3. Health Education–methods.
4. Life Style. W 85 L7223 2008]

RA776.9.L56 2008
613–dc22

2007049689

A catalogue record for this book is available from the British Library.

Set in 10.5/12.5 pt Palatino by Newgen Imaging Systems (P) Ltd, Chennai, India
Printed and bound in Singapore by Markono Print Media Pte Ltd

1 2008

Contents

Contributors

Jamie Bell, MSc, MCSP SRP, BSc (Hons) With an early career background as a physiotherapist in sports medicine, this author is now appointed as senior lecturer in physiotherapy and director of the Spinal Research Group at Leeds Metropolitan University. He is also a member of the Spinal Research Unit at the University of Huddersfield, where he is now completing his PhD, investigating the impact of work-related biomechanical and psychosocial factors on low back pain and related sickness absence. He has presented at numerous international scientific conferences, and is regularly invited to review articles for scientific journals.

Gill Coverdale, MSc, BSc (Hons), RGN, Cert Ed Gill initially trained as an Registered Nurse before having her children. For the majority of her career, she worked in the community first within the district nursing team and then as a school nursing specialist practitioner for 14 years working with children and young people and their families. She has experience as a practice nurse too. She completed her Cert Ed in 1995 in order to enhance her health promotion skills and knowledge. She completed a first degree in Specialist Community Nursing, and then went on to teach first in the FE sector and then in the higher education sector in 2001 leading the school nursing pathway of the Specialist Community Public Health Nursing Degree programme. She is a member of the Advancing Health Care Practice Group at Leeds Metropolitan University. She recently completed a masters degree in public health and carried out research on public health nursing. She is a member of the expert advisor group at the Department of Health for children of school age and contributed to two recent government publications. Her research and practice interest lies in public health of children/young people and in inter-professional learning across traditional boundaries.

Jim McKenna PhD, MPhil, PGCE is Professor of Physical Activity and Health at Leeds Metropolitan University. He has published over 40 peer reviewed papers, many in the field of physical activity promotion in medical and workplace settings. In his current post he is leading the research centre for Active Lifestyles, which houses over 15 actively researching academics and a number of PhD students. He was a scientific contributor to two chapters in the Chief Medical Officer's Report (2004) and has co-edited *Perspectives on Health and Exercise* (2003). He is an active reviewer for 12 peer reviewed journals and for five international grant-awarding groups and has been a postgraduate external examiner for six UK and Irish universities.

Stephen Paul, MSc Psychological Counselling, Post Grad Cert Ed, DipClient-centred Psychotherapy, Dip Business and Executive Coaching, BA (Hons), Cert Special Needs Education, Stephen Paul is currently director for the Centre for Psychological Therapies at Leeds Metropolitan University. Stephen is a psychotherapist with over 30 years of practitioner experience within mental health with adult and child/adolescent-aged clients. He was previously the head of a special school for children with emotional and behavioural difficulties. He has particular interests and expertise in existential, humanistic and transpersonal psychologies, client-centred psychotherapy, spirituality and group therapy. He has studied extensively in areas of psychological counselling, teaching, business and executive coaching. He currently has a book *The Therapeutic Relationship: Themes and Perspectives* in print. He has taught courses in therapeutic skills to a range of health and social care professionals and has led courses in counselling and psychotherapy since 1992.

Sue Pemberton, MSc, Bsc (Hons), Dip COT Sue is a qualified occupational therapist who was involved in setting up a clinical service in Leeds for people with chronic fatigue syndrome in 1990, one of the first National Health Service clinics specifically for the condition. She wrote the original therapy programme and has continued to work clinically with the service throughout its history, despite having a broad career in mental health management. Sue is currently the clinical champion for the condition for the North, East and West Yorkshire area and contributes to collaborative work nationally in this field. She is the only consultant occupational therapist working in CFS/ME (Chronic Fatigue Syndrome/Myalgic Encephalomyelitis) in the country, speaking regularly at national conferences on the condition and contributing to the national training of health professionals.

Bill Penson, BSc (Hons) Psychology, BSc (Hons) Psychosocial Interventions for Severe Mental Illness, PGCHE Bill is a senior lecturer in Mental Health and has worked at Leeds Metropolitan University since 2003. His practice background is mental health social care and the third sector, residential and community. He has particular interests in working with psychosis, the therapeutic relationship and education for support workers. Bill is involved in a range of workforce development activities for mental health practitioners including consultation, training and supervision. He has presented work at a number of conferences about training practitioners in evidence-based practice and using narratives in learning. In his spare time, he is a fencing coach and has recently published an article looking at the use of cognitive therapy models in understanding a fencer's performance.

Pinki Sahota, PhD, BSc, RD, RPHNut Pinki Sahota is Reader in Childhood Obesity at Leeds Metropolitan University. She is also a state registered dietician and a registered public health nutritionist with over 17 years experience in community dietetics. In her role as a community dietician, she has worked within the primary care setting and was involved in running dietetic clinics for a range of patients with diet-related conditions including obesity, hyperlipidaemia, and diabetes including the development of appropriate diet sheets and resources. She has been involved in setting up new multidisciplinary primary care services including primary-care-based diabetic clinics for patients with Type II diabetes and weight reducing clinics. Dr Sahota has delivered training sessions on management of diabetes, hyperlipidaemia and obesity for primary care staff including, specifically, practice nurses and general practitioners. She is currently involved in research in the management of adult obesity in primary care. The study involved the development, implementation and evaluation of a practice nurse training programme including a resource manual. This work was commissioned by Leeds PCT and is currently undergoing evaluation. Dr Sahota is committed to improving community-based interventions aimed at the prevention and treatment of obesity both through her research and her teaching.

Dawn Taylor, Msc Social Research and Evaluation, RGN, PGCE Dawn originally qualified at an RGN, but went on to qualify as a midwife and a health visitor. She has worked in many different areas as a health visitor and gained a wide community experience whilst doing a counselling course and practice teacher and assessors course. Her last four years as a health visitor were spent on Secondment to region working as a CESDI (Confidential Enquiry into Stillbirths and Deaths in Infancy) health visitor. During this period, she also completed an MSc in social research and evaluation at Huddersfield University and her dissertation was a comparative study of birth plans within three hospitals in West Yorkshire. She is currently working as Health Visitor Course Leader at Leeds Metropolitan University. Dawn has a keen interest in sudden infant death and bereavement counselling. Her other interests lie within public health and non-medical prescribing.

Miranda Thew, MSc Health Professional Education, BHSc (Hons), Dip COT, Cert Management, PGCHE Miranda has had a varied clinical background as an occupational therapist within mental health for nearly 20 years, but more lately within liaison psychiatry. She worked clinically and was clinical team manager for a chronic fatigue syndrome service for a number of years. She regularly presents at national and local events regarding current occupational therapy practice. Whilst working in a community mental health team, she completed her masters degree; her dissertation was a randomised controlled treatment trial of a relaxation regime with irritable bowel syndrome patients within a gastroenterology clinic. She is currently employed at Leeds Metropolitan University as senior lecturer in occupational science and occupational therapy. She is completing a PhD which explores student lifestyle choice and influences on health. Miranda also contributes to the university staff development programme on lifestyle management and well-being.

Fiona Wondergem, MSc, BSc (Hons), RGN, RSCN, PGDip Health Visiting Fiona is a practising health visitor at Kirklees PCT and also a part-time lecturer at the University of Huddersfield. Fiona's MSc dissertation in Public Health discussed the need to provide more inclusive services for breastfeeding women. She also has a professional interest in child development and parenting skills. Fiona has also worked as editor of the Journal of Community Nursing for the past 17 years and is a member of the Guild of Health Writers. Married with three children she enjoys travelling, horse riding, reading and sleeping.

Acknowledgements

We would like to thank the contributors for their commitment and passion for their subjects. Without you, this book would lack the breadth and depth of experience and relevance.

To the commissioning editor and her team, thank you for your patience, support and expert guidance in making the seemingly impossible a reality.

Overwhelmingly, we must acknowledge our friends and family, especially Isabella who in her first few weeks of life, has had to compete for Mummy's attention with three siblings and a computer!

Introduction

Miranda Thew and Jim McKenna

Health and social care professionals are either directly providing lifestyle advice or supporting healthy lifestyles as an add-on to their usual span of skills and specialities. Even though recent government documentation has been devised on specific lifestyle areas, such as increasing exercise (Department of Health, 2004), for most staff such documents do little to address the span of lifestyle concerns. This resource, written by professionals with extensive experience and research in various lifestyle elements, provides pertinent, accessible, practical, and wide-ranging information in the areas that dominate in therapy sessions. Each chapter outlines the current research base to support lifestyle advice, supported by resources that can be distributed to clients. These resources include photocopyable handouts, exercises and activities with links to relevant associations for the more complex issues. An important feature of the text is a supporting chapter (Chapter 1) detailing the elements that underpin personal change.

The chapter topics have been carefully selected to represent the typical issues encountered in practice and they cover the elements of life that can be deleterious to well-being. There are sections on fatigue, sleep and stress management (relaxation), all of which are influential in a number of severely debilitating diseases and illnesses. Lower back pain, fatigue and stress are common problems in their own right and account for large proportions of primary clinic attendances as well as subsequent demands on health care services. The importance of healthy family relationships, another focus of governmental policy, is supported here with chapters on parenting young children and teenagers. Obesity is now of such national importance that there are numerous health care initiatives attempting to address the lifestyle factors causing it. High blood pressure is a significant risk factor in coronary heart disease, yet is readily treatable largely with lifestyle strategies. Work/life balance can lead to numerous conflicts which contribute to dissatisfaction with life. These can lead to unhelpful behaviours that subsequently have an impact on well-being and health. All these factors can contribute to inappropriate coping behaviours (such as alcohol abuse), thus leading to further lifestyle problems.

Why we need healthy lifestyles

It is well reported that a healthy lifestyle can reduce the morbidity and mortality of life-threatening conditions such as cancer and coronary heart disease (Chiuve *et al.*, 2006). Although technological advances in medical testing and treatment have increased life expectancy, the relative costs to health care are now being realised; yet government objectives and investment are lacking in addressing fundamental lifestyle risk factors (Wanless, 2004). Indeed, projected quality-adjusted life year expectancy can increase by providing lifestyle management programmes for preventable diseases, thereby making them a cost-effective intervention (Graves *et al.*, 2006). Beyond immediate remedial costs, preventable ill-health also adds to national budgets in many other ways, including exaggerated use of health and social care services through stress and various forms of substance abuse (Goldberg, 1999).

Recent research by Developing Patient Partnerships (DPP) found that health professionals working in primary care believe there is a greater need for health information for their patients than ever before and that GP practices should provide this information (DPP, 2007). Even in prestigious professional journals such as the *British Medical Journal*, evidence-based papers are consulted less often than those providing expert narrative (Loke and Derry, 2003). This suggests that professionals prefer resources that help them to learn more practical and clinical skills than to hear about complex research-based outcomes.

Time to move beyond 'common-sense' advice

Although 'lifestyle' is central to many health programmes, including cardiac rehabilitation (Eckel, 2006), cancer therapy (Rock and Demark-Wahnefried, 2002) and drug and alcohol rehabilitation, there remains a need for a single up-to-date and accessible general lifestyle resource that goes beyond the common-sense advice that is likely to prevail in daily practice. It has been generally found that people value lifestyle advice from primary care practitioners (Richmond *et al.*, 1996). In addition, a large-scale study (McAvoy *et al.*, 1999) found that general practitioners (GPs) are confident in pointing out the risks to health from lifestyle behaviours. However, they were less confident that they could provide the necessary information, or had the skills and training to facilitate change in their patients. It is also clear that many professionals know little of how to deliver lifestyle support to reluctant, resistant or even belligerent clients, with few professionals reporting recent training in up-to-date behaviour-change approaches (McKenna and Vernon, 2004).

For these reasons, having an accessible, informative guide, which acts as an incentive for further promotion of lifestyle change, will be a boon for most health care professionals. Whether individuals want to be faced with the inconvenient truth that their lifestyle is killing them or not, it is down to local, accessible professionals to feel comfortable to impart sensible, evidenced advice to enable long-standing change and facilitate better client outcomes. Even specialists will benefit from the text, which will help them to support their delivery of usual care with supportive behaviour change theory and expert-developed, ready-prepared client handouts.

Ultimately, healthy longevity lies within the capacities of most people; essentially, it is their daily life habits which need to be addressed, and it is the role of professionals to help adults to change those habits that are at the root of their difficulties. By providing health and social care professionals with the tools to facilitate life changes, the timeliness of this manual could hardly be better.

Note on terminology

The term 'client' has been used throughout the book to indicate service user, client and patient.

References

Chiuve, S. E., McCullough, M. L., Sacks, F. M. and Rimm, E. B. (2006). Healthy lifestyle factors in the primary prevention of coronary heart disease among men: benefits among users and nonusers of lipid-lowering and antihypertensive medications. *Circulation*, 114: 160–167.

Department of Health (2004). *Physical Activity, Health Improvement and Prevention. At Least Five a Week.* London, Department of Health.

DPP (2007). Health professionals desperate for health information for their patients. Developing Patient Partnerships. http://www.dpp.org.uk. Retrieved 2 October 2007.

Eckel, R. H. (2006). Preventive cardiology by lifestyle intervention: opportunity and/or challenge? Presidential Address at the 2005 American Heart Association Scientific Sessions. *Circulation,* 113: 2657–2661.

Graves, N., McKinnon, L., Reeves, M., Scuffham, P., Gordon, L. and Eakin, E. (2006). Cost-effectiveness analyses and modelling the lifetime costs and benefits of health-behaviour interventions. *Chronic Illness,* 2: 97–107.

Goldberg, D. (1999). The management of anxious depression in primary care. *Journal of Clinical Psychiatry*, 60: 39–44.

Loke, Y. K. and Derry, S. (2003). Does anybody read 'evidence based' articles? *BMC Medical Research Methodology,* **3:** 616–621.

McAvoy, B. R., Kaner, E. F., Lock, C. A., Heather, N. and Gilvarry, E. (1999). Our healthier nation: are general practitioners willing and able to deliver? A survey of attitudes to and involvement in health promotion and lifestyle counselling. *British Journal of General Practice,* 49: 187–190.

McKenna, J. and Vernon, M. (2004). How general practitioners promote 'lifestyle' physical activity. *Patient Education and Counselling*, 54: 101–106.

Richmond, R., Kehoe, L., Heather, N., Wodak, A. and Webster, I. (1996). General practitioners' promotion of healthy lifestyles: what patients think. *Australian and New Zealand Journal of Public Health,* 20: 195–200.

Rock, C. L. and Demark-Wahnefried, W. (2002). Can lifestyle modification increase survival in women diagnosed with breast cancer? *Journal of Nutrition*, 132: 504–509.

Wanless, D. (2004). *Securing Good Health for the Whole Population: Final Report*. London, HM Treasury.

Section A
HEALTHY LIFESTYLES

1. *Creating the Opportunity for Change*

Stephen Paul and Bill Penson

Introduction

This chapter deals in working with clients to enable them to achieve personal and psychological change. Effective change can be facilitated by the development of positive helping relationships. The helping professional can refine the way they engage with the client to maximise their outcome with the client. This will not simply be achieved by 'telling' the client what to do, but by working with them to help them become motivated and maintain a plan of action.

There is wealth of evidence which demonstrates the importance of the therapeutic relationship being central in helping settings (Lambert, 2003). Whilst many health and social care professionals cannot expect to have the time or resources to build deep relationships with their clients, it is possible to create the conditions for effective individual change within short time frames. The health care practitioner, be they a nurse, doctor, physiotherapist, dietician or other professional working with a wide range of different issues from sleep management to pain control, can develop interpersonal strategies to achieve good results. By harnessing the individual's motivation and offering structure and focus, the professional can work with the client to achieve practical change.

Interpersonal or counselling skills can be developed by all health care professionals (Gable, 2007). Research has demonstrated a clear connection between effective helping relationships and positive outcomes (Hargie and Dickson, 2004) and this chapter will consider:

- The context in which the client and the helping professional meet.
- An individual's internal psychological factors including his/her motivation for change.

- Creating an effective therapeutic relationship.
- Enabling action for change.

We aim to equip the practitioner to work with their client towards recognisably achievable goals.

Context and practice rationale

It is hoped that by the end of this section you will be thinking about how to offer a rationale for your application of new knowledge and articulating the clients' opportunity for change. However, this needs to be situated in a broader practice context. This is because most health and social care practitioners work within a team context and whilst there are varying degrees of autonomy and lone working most will be working alongside others. Besides other professionals, there may also be contact with the client's family, friends and carers. Whitlock *et al.* (2002) recommend that practitioners take an 'ecological view' with a client, and understand them within their social, economic and political context. Clearly, there are a range of skills and knowledge required on the part of the practitioner to change their focus between individual, family, team and organisational contexts for service delivery. With this in mind, it is important to reflect on the importance of the setting and context of personal practice. Taking each in turn, the following sections describe a number of 'locations' where client work may be situated, with brief explanation and questions to guide reflection.

Policy drivers and case management

There are likely to be policy drivers both national and local that influence and direct an individual practitioner, both professionally and in service provision. These can offer a useful backdrop to understanding interventions and in explaining these to colleagues and clients. In Advice box 1.1 you will find some questions that will guide your thinking on relevant current policy, they can provide some help in understanding barriers to innovative practice.

With most health and social care professionals working in multi-disciplinary teams and across agency boundaries, it is important to understand how practitioner interventions fit within a team approach and particularly where there are complex or long-term needs within local care pathways. You may well be working as case manager for clients and if not, then liaising closely with the case manager. Good interdisciplinary working is viewed as essential in a range of settings and is driven by various policy documents. See Advice box 1.2 for tips on working well within a case management framework.

Evidence-based practice (EBP) and value-based practice (VBP)

Increasingly, a range of professionals are being required to demonstrate a clarity in their skill deployment and a contemporary knowledge base that is made up of both evidence-based approaches and technologies, and a clear value base (for instance, National Health Service [NHS] staff through the Knowledge/Skills Framework and National Occupational Standards [DH, 2003]). In addition to their professional role, practitioners are also obliged to be a learner and implementer of evidence. Sometimes working to an evidence base can feel at a distance to the human contact of your role, and indeed evidence suggests that research findings can be difficult to implement (Rolfe, 1998). Figure 1.1 shows how Bury (2002) has articulated the role of EBP.

This model is clearly interactional and requires the practitioner to be aware of their own internal influences, for instance, beliefs about how the world should be, how a client ought to behave and what is good for the client. In addition, there may be more socially and

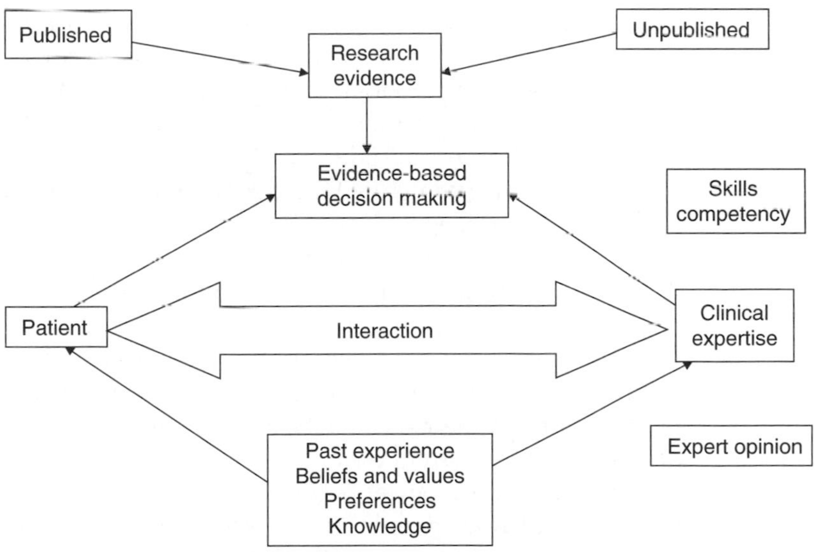

Fig. 1.1 Evidence-based practice and decision making (Bury, 2002).

culturally bound meanings and beliefs relating to illness, gender, sexuality, disability, race and age. A self-reflective style in combination with an appropriate value base can help the practitioner understand what they bring to each contact they have, and is therefore self-supervising in that respect (Kottler and Jones, 2003). Bolton (2005) highlights the importance of reflective practice and provides a helpful guide to thinking and writing reflectively.

Similarly, the client brings an internal world that interacts with the intervention, practitioner and the setting. At heart, Bury (2002) is suggesting that there is a dynamism in EBP going beyond the application of research to a clinical problem.

Taking a psychological view

This section introduces the idea that to engage and optimise change for clients, practitioners need to engage with the inner mental world and understanding of the client.

Clients and their families will be making sense of their health and health problems in many ways, sometimes termed 'lay views'. To the practitioner, these strategies or lay models can appear and be counterproductive. However, clients and their families will demonstrate an effortful process of coping with good use of strategies and innovative ways of managing. Practitioners need to take an increasingly sophisticated view of coping, which goes beyond the scope of this chapter. Part of this will be accepting and working with where the client 'is at' in the present. In health care settings, we may be more orientated to personal stories of coping and restitution (Frank, 1995) which may not reflect how the clients view their story and indeed how it may unfold. Practitioner's beliefs about the role of coping in recovery may well be overstated, as demonstrated in the review by Petticrew *et al.* (2002) on recovery with cancer, wherein recurrence was not impacted on by coping, despite indications that it does in small studies, and they recommend that people should not be pressurised into particular ways of coping.

Service delivery is often set up to deal with problems and needs, not necessarily attuned to the strengths, resources and competence of the client and their social network. We will return to the relevance of understanding strengths and resources.

Taking a psychological view would involve understanding the mechanics of how people think (information processing, problem solving, etc.) and how they think in terms of their views (internal models, biases, experience) and their emotional world. There are many elements to these areas including motivation, a client's locus of control, self-efficacy, learning capacity and skills, values and social learning. We have only considered psychological elements although clearly the social and biological also have enormous influence and constant interaction. Discursive psychologists would claim that there is a need to understand illness both socially and within time, highlighting the limits of a cognitive interpretation (Marks *et al.*, 2005). This highlights the complexity and interconnectedness of the psychological, social, temporal and biological world in working with change, and thus the need to understand and engage the client as expert in their experience (refer back to Figure 1.1 for a model of how this might interact). The notion of expert patient, and its relationship to patient centred care and user involvement, is widely believed to be a significant ethos for adoption in health and social care whilst acknowledging that this is also fraught with tensions and barriers (Wilson, 2001; Tattersall, 2002).

Increasingly, health and social care professionals are encouraged to develop their psychological mindedness. This can quite simply be understood as an interest and concern within the inner world of others, thinking and emotional, and having the corresponding skills and knowledge that allows you to make sense of this inner world. This may represent a considerable personal and professional challenge which may be best met by adopting a framework or model to work within. There is a range of psychotherapeutic, health promotion and adult learning models, with training often readily available, which can be drawn on (for instance, cognitive-behavioural, solution-focused and person-centred models).

Engaging with a client's way of viewing their world and their problems is immensely important. Lay beliefs can affect a range of behaviours from engagement with health professionals to adherence to treatment (Heurtin-Roberts and Reisin, 1992; Walter *et al.*, 2004). If we accept the potency of some lay views of health problems, we then have to engage with the complex interaction of variables that perpetuate such beliefs, be they individual psychological variables or demographic factors such as poverty (Marks *et al.*, 2005).

Antonovsky (1979) suggests that health experiences are on a continuum. We are not healthy *or* diseased but rather on a continuum between these two poles, and we can move on this continuum. He goes on to suggest that there are factors that enable people to shift towards the health end of the continuum. These factors are threefold: how comprehensible, meaningful and manageable the problem is to the person. In using this model to understand how to engender change in clients, we engage immediately with the idea that their internal world has a lot to do with how healthy they can make themselves. This also immediately suggests the value of interventions based on giving information (considering both form and accessibility [French and Swain, 2004]), solving problems and being goal orientated (Free, 2007). Antonovsky goes on to suggest that people have resources they can apply in weathering setbacks and dealing with problems, and in combination with their views and thoughts about their lives, they have a sense of coherence around their health. By extension, to help clients gain a sense of coherence and move towards health, they will need to make sense of their problems, understand and give meaning to them, and have the resources to mobilise and manage them.

Psychological ways of helping tend to fall towards two approaches:

1. *Changes in thinking and feeling*: Some manner of helping process engages the client in articulating their feelings and thinking around a problem area with a view to venting and expressing, and then to problem solving or resolution. The thinking occurs prior to behaviour change.
2. *Changes in behaviour*: Changes in activity are enacted with corresponding reflection on the activity. Thinking and feeling change as a result of a different actual experience. Often activity is graded, rehearsed, practised and linked to rewards and incentives.

Most change models appear to start with one of these and will encourage the shift to the other during the change process. This is a useful notion in locating practice: where do you start in your interventions and which is the most helpful place to begin?

Working therapeutically with motivation

This section explores the importance of client motivation in achieving their results and offers strategies to enable effective work with adults. Researched motivational approaches that are relevant in both health/social care practice and in psychological coaching in sport and business are used (Gallwey, 1974, 1985, 2000; Bluckert, 2006).

Evidence suggests that with the right conditions individuals will seek to better themselves of their own accord (Elliott *et al.*, 2004). The helping professional therefore, by laying the foundations for a positive helping relationship, can work together with the individual's motivation on a commonly agreed plan of action. The focus on easily achievable, positive actions will enable the individual to move from an inhibiting situation towards action and empowerment. It is therefore important for the helping professional to work with the individual towards his/her chosen goals.

Motivation can be applied to all areas of human action. Understanding motivation is, in fact, key to models of 'health behaviour' such as the 'health belief model', where health seeking is based on an interaction of four main elements: perceived susceptibility to a problem, perceived seriousness of the consequences of the problem, perceived benefits of an action and perceived barriers to action (Nutbeam and Harris, 1999). Alongside this, Motivational Theory is based on the premise that the individual will seek to satisfy his/her needs. This may be:

1. *The satisfaction of basic needs* such as eating, drinking and keeping warm.
2. *The need to reduce or eliminate painful experiences* such as anxiety provoking situations or depressing thoughts.
3. *The need to experience fulfilment* such as good relationships or the enjoyment of music or sport.

Maslow's (1999) 'hierarchy of human needs theory' is one of the most commonly used models of motivation. Maslow's research and theories have been applied to many areas of human development (Hoffman, 1999). Motivational counselling and interviewing have been developed in many areas of health and social care and have been proven effective in work with addictions, in health promotion and in other settings (e.g. Resnicow *et al.*, 2002).

Maslow believed that human needs are motivational in that unsatisfied needs can affect behaviour whereas needs that are satisfied do not. He proposed a hierarchy of needs from the basic physiological needs to the higher-order aesthetic and fulfilment needs. Figure 1.2 demonstrates original needs listed from basic to most complex.

More recently, psychologists and therapists have believed that working with all parts of the individual enables those parts which may be stuck or unresolved to move and change.

So rather than treat human development as a pyramid to climb or a stepladder of goals, it is more helpful to consider an individual's needs, wants and desires to be part of a *gestalt* or whole in which all parts feed into each other like parts of a jigsaw. Sometimes by working with the pieces around a difficult area the individual can see the problem and the missing piece more easily. In effect, by working

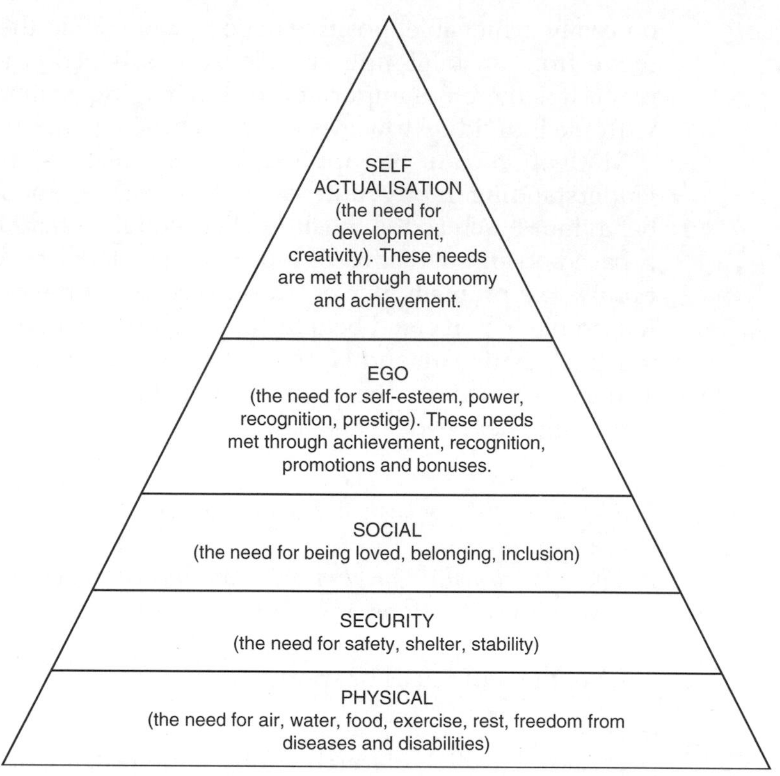

Fig. 1.2 An illustration of Maslow's hierarchy of needs. Adapted from Maslow (1943, 1999).

with all areas of your client's life you can help the client to make the changes themselves in the particular problem area; that is, someone struggling to stop smoking may find the will power to do so when they are fulfilling themselves in other areas of their life.

It is helpful therefore to help harness the individual's motivation to change by helping her/him create a template for change. Handout 1.1 offers a three-stage strategy to help your client review their present situation.

There are other ways that have enabled people to make life changes that have been developed by the psychologist Kurt Lewin and the coach and writer Timothy Gallwey. Lewin (1943) developed what he called a force-field analysis (www.mindtools.com/pages/article/newTED_06.htm). He proposed that individuals will choose to move towards the best results for them but in certain circumstances will be impeded by restraining forces. If any individual can work to reduce the influence of these restraining forces, he/she can more easily achieve his/her potential (see Advice box 1.4).

We are capable therefore of achieving what our inner obstacles allow us to. Remove internal obstacles and our performance develops to meet our potential. Similarly, by reducing the power of obstacles in relation to any task, we face the potential to successfully achieve our task.

Lewin (1946) through his research, created the fundamental observation that the Behaviour of a person (B) is a Function (f) of the interaction of that person's Personality (P) and the present human and physical Environment (E). This formula $B = f(P, E)$ is important in that it locates the experiences and behaviour of the individual in the present. The individual can therefore make significant life changes without undergoing in-depth long-term psychological therapy. By changing the environment the individuals can change the way they think and feel.

Timothy Gallwey developed the notion of the inner game (1974). He said we have an outer game and an inner game. The outer game is our behaviour and the circumstances we face. The inner game is our internal world and there is always an inner game playing in our mind whatever is happening on the outside. Building on the work of Lewin, he formulated the notion,

$$\text{Performance} = \text{potential minus interference, or } P = p - i.$$

According to this formula, performance can be enhanced either by *growing* potential or by *decreasing* interference. All clinicians can relate anecdotes of clients who outwardly seem well equipped to make life changes but seem unable to achieve their goals (see Advice box 1.5).

Another approach that has been developed in psychological, sport and business coaching is the GROW model (Whitmore, 2002). The model has four stages: Goal – Current Reality – Options – Way forward (Advice box 1.6). Variations of this model are most commonly used in motivational coaching. Handout 1.2 can be used with clients.

Building a therapeutic relationship

In the latter part of the twentieth century, health care professionals were criticised for poor interpersonal skills as the traditional emphasis was on the professional as a diagnoser and expert administrator of treatment (Hargie and Dickson, 2004). There have been changes in recent times with courses on interpersonal and counselling skills being introduced into professional training.

Whilst each client is unique and idiosyncratic, the therapeutic relationship is central to personal change in helping settings (Beutler *et al.*, 2003). A wealth of research (Roth and Fonagy, 2004) indicates that three key factors in building effective helping relationships are:

1. *Empathy towards the client.* The attempt by the practitioner to really understand the client, his/her position and world view, without interpretation, is considered central.
2. *Genuineness and authenticity on the part of the practitioner.* If the client perceives the practitioner as a human being not hiding behind a professional façade and genuinely seeking to help, research tells us that clients will find this authenticity truly helpful. The practitioner is not required to disengage from their professional role but to be present and engage actively to help the client. The client seeks help for themselves, and it may not be helpful to work with them as a diagnostic category.
3. *Acceptance by the practitioner of the client and his/her world view.* Here the evidence is that clients, who do not feel judged or treated as an object by the professional, report their experiences positively. This attitude may also be considered *prizing* or *valuing*.

There is significant evidence to suggest that the wholehearted application of the above attitudes, in themselves, lead to positively reported outcomes (Bozarth, 1998). Furthermore, it is important that these attitudes are communicated to and received by the client. Your clients will not know your values and qualities unless these are communicated in your behaviour.

Evidence suggests that where clients do not feel positive about a helping professional they will not return to the helping agency. It is therefore important to create the right climate for your client to feel understood and valued.

The role of brief contacts

As previously mentioned, often practitioners have time constrictions in their face-to-face contacts, so making the most of such time is essential. Structure-, focus- and goal-orientated approaches will optimise contacts. Strange *et al.* (2002) discuss the benefits and feasibility of 'one minute for prevention' where the practitioner gives a focused 1 minute health promoting intervention within a longer (but still brief) contact.

In a relatively brief period of contact, the individual can be invited to review the fulfilment of needs in all areas of life till now and identify their aspirations. The individual can then put in place a simple and practical plan for the fulfilment of needs in one or more areas. This will then enable a snowballing of positive activity, called the 'snowball effect'. See Handout 1.1 for a 'life review' activity.

Structure and focus

In the previous sections we discussed engaging the practitioner in understanding the psychological world of the client as a means to understanding how to optimise change. If we return briefly to Figure 1.1 we see that the practitioner has a very significant role in this too and perhaps the most useful way to view the promotion of change is that the process is interactional: client with practitioner. As a result the practitioner needs to be motivated, communicate values, articulate working models, communicate hope and optimism. This moves practice away from 'doing to' to 'doing with'.

Padesky quotes a number of studies which suggest that positive outcomes in therapy are linked to the degree of structure and focus, which in turn is best articulated through understanding the therapeutic alliance. Therapeutic alliance is where there is a positive bond between the client and practitioner; there is agreement on goals and agreement on tasks (Safran and Muran, 2000). These three components are very helpful to the practitioner in reflecting on problems in the process of change, and we would recommend that whenever the practitioner encounters problems in working with a client's change, they return to therapeutic alliance (see Advice box 1.4).

The advantages of structure and focus include:

- Making optimal use of time together.
- Being entirely transparent and collaborative in negotiating your joint efforts.
- Negotiating 'homework' tasks between meetings to facilitate generalisation of new learning and increase a sense of autonomy.
- More easily predicting where the work will lead.
- More easily measuring progress and outcomes.
- Locating setbacks within a larger process.

The Cognitive Therapy Scale is a validated tool for measuring deployment of therapy skills both generally and with specificity to the cognitive therapy model. Some of the subscales particularly address structure and focus including agenda setting, eliciting feedback and interpersonal effectiveness. This scale can be found at www.beckinstitute.com.

Whitlock *et al.* (2002) recommend a 5 A's approach that can offer a useful structure to health promoting activities, especially where contact time is brief. These are *Assess* (health, risks, factors affecting choice, goals), *Advise* (education and information giving), *Agree* (collaboration on goals and methods tailored to the client), *Assist* (supporting behaviour change through skills training, building confidence, considering social/environmental support, etc.) and *Arrange* (follow-up, reviewing and changing plans, offering ongoing support). The 5 A's model is used frequently in smoking cessation work and can be used in combination with other models for chronic conditions (Glasgow and Emmons, 2007). Studies indicate that practitioners may need support in implementing Assist and Arrange which are less well delivered than the other As (Yusem *et al.*, 2004; Glasgow and Emmons, 2007).

Identifying problems can be reformulated into having goals. So if the problem is not having meaningful activity (this is difficult to do something with) the goal can be to seek appropriate meaningful activity (far easier to work towards).

In setting goals, you will need to make sure that you are collaborating and these goals are those of the client. If there are problems in doing this, then you may wish to return to reflect on the therapeutic alliance. In Handout 1.3, you can see the Strengths model case management assessment (based on the concept described in Morgan, 1996). This is a very useful exercise to undertake because not only does it elicit strengths and resources which can be overlooked in people with health problems, but it also forms the basis of goal setting. In addition, when the practitioner discusses hopes for the future genuinely, this communicates optimism.

Goal setting is best when the goals are SMART: specific, measurable, achievable, realistic and timed. This pneumonic provides a useful checklist to compare and construct the goals being articulated.

Conclusion

This chapter introduced the context for change including the team and service context, and set the scene for a psychological view. Given both the limits practitioners often experience in practice and also the importance of clients being autonomous in their health, important factors were considered in engendering an ethos of change. Practitioners need to be psychologically minded, interpersonally effective and be able to communicate optimism when working with a client. The interaction between good use of EBP and expertise, dovetailing this with policy, combined with interpersonal effectiveness makes for a potent blend. Many of the factors outlined are useful for clients and applicable for practitioners themselves. The forming of a sound relationship and alliance remains at the heart of the process for change.

References

Antonovsky, A. (1979). *Health, Stress & Coping*. London, Jossey-Bass.

Beutler, L. E., Malik, M., Alimohamed, S. *et al.* (2003). Therapist variables. In Lambert, M. J. (ed.) *Bergin & Garfield's Handbook of Psychotherapy and Behaviour Change*, 5th edition. New York, Wiley, pp. 207–226

Bluckert, P. (2006). *Psychological Dimensions to Executive Coaching*. Oxford, OUP.

Bolton, G. (2005). *Reflective Practice: Writing & Professional Development*. London, Sage.

Bozarth, J. D. (1998). *Person-Centred Therapy: A Revolutionary Paradigm*. Ross-on-Wye, PCCS Books.

Bury, T. (2002). Evidence based health care explained. In Bury, T. and Mead, J. (eds) *Evidence-based Healthcare: A Practical Guide for Therapists*. Oxford, Butterworth Heinemann, p. 10.

Department of Health (2003). *The NHS Knowledge & Skills Framework (NHS KSF) and Development Review Guidance*. http://www.dh.gov.uk/en/Publicationsandstatistics/Publications/PublicationsPolicyAndGuidance/DH_4009176. Accessed 18 May 2007.

Elliott, R., Greenberg, L. S. and Lietaer, G. (2004). Research in experiential therapies. In Lambert, M. J. (ed.) *Bergin & Garfield's Handbook of Psychotherapy and Behaviour Change*, 5th edition. New York, Wiley, pp. 493–440.

Frank, A. W. (1995). *The Wounded Storyteller*. Chicago, University of Chicago Press.

Free, M. L. (2007). *Cognitive Therapy in Groups*. Chichester, Wiley.

French, S. and Swain, J. (2004). Disability and communication: listening is not enough. In Robb, M., Barret, S., Komaromy, C. and Rodgers, A. (eds) *Communication, Relationships and Care: A Reader*. London, Routledge, pp. 220–234.

Gable, J. (2007). *Counselling Skills for Dieticians*. Oxford, Blackwell.

Gallwey, T. W. (1974). *The Inner Game of Tennis*. New York, Random House.

Gallwey, T. W. (1985). *Inner Game of Winning*. New York, Random House.

Gallwey, T. W. (2000). *The Inner Game of Work – Focus, Learning, Pleasure, and Mobility in the Workplace*. New York, Random House.

Glasgow, R. E. and Emmons, K. M. (2007). How can we increase translation of research into practice? Types of evidence needed. *Annual Review of Public Health*, 28: 413–433.

Hargie, O. and Dickson, D. (2004). *Skilled Interpersonal Communication Research, Theory and Practice*, 4th edition. Hove, Routledge.

Heurtin-Roberts, S. and Reisin, E. (1992). The relation of culturally influenced lay models of hypertension to compliance with treatment. *American Journal of Hypertension*, 5: 787–792.

Hoffman, E. (1999). *Right to be Human: Biography of Abraham Maslow*, 2nd edition. New York, McGraw-Hill Education.

Kottler, J. A. and Jones, W. P. (2003). *Doing Better: Improving Clinical Skills and Professional Competence*. Hove, Brunner-Routledge.

Lambert, J. M. (ed.) (2003). *Bergin & Garfield's Handbook of Psychotherapy and Behaviour Change*, 5th edition. New York, Wiley.

Lewin, K. (1943). Defining the 'Field at a Given Time'. *Psychological Review*, 50: 292–310. Republished in *Resolving Social Conflicts & Field Theory in Social Science*. Washington, DC, American Psychological Association, 1997.

Lewin, K. (1946). Behavior and development as a function of the total situation. In Carmichael, L. (ed.) *Manual of Child Psychology*. New York, John Wiley & Sons.

Marks, D. F., Murray, M., Evans, B., Willig, C., Woodall, C. and Sykes, C. M. (2005). *Health Psychology: Theory, Research & Practice*. London, Sage.

Maslow, A. H. (1943). A theory of human motivation. *Psychological Review*, 50: 370–396.

Maslow, A. H. (1999). *Toward's a Psychology of Being*, 3rd edition. New York, Wiley.

Morgan, S. (1996). *Helping Relationships in Mental Health*. London, Chapman & Hall.

Neenan, M. and Dryden, W. (2001). *Learning from Errors in Rational Emotive Behaviour Therapy*. London, Whurr Publishers.

Nutbeam, D. and Harris, E. (1999). *Theory in a Nutshell: A Guide to Health Promotion Theory*. London, McGraw-Hill.

Petticrew, M., Bell, R. and Hunter, D. (2002). Influence of psychological coping on survival and recurrence in people with cancer: systematic review. *British Medical Journal*, 325: 1066–1069.

Resnicow, K., DiIorio, C., Soet, J. E., Ernst, D., Borrelli, B. and Hecht, J. (2002). Motivational interviewing in health promotion: it sounds like something is changing. *Health Psychology*, 21: 444–451.

Rolfe, G. (1998). The theory-practice gap in nursing: from research based practice to practitioner-based research. *Journal of Advanced Nursing*, 28: 672–679.

Roth, A. and Fonagy, P. (2004). *What Works for Whom? A Critical Review of Psychotherapy Research*, 2nd edition. New York, Guilford Press.

Safran, J. D. and Muran, J. C. (2000). *Negotiating the Therapeutic Alliance: A Relational Treatment Guide*. London, The Guilford Press.

Strange, K. C., Woolf, S. H. and Gjeltema, K. (2002). One minute for prevention. The power of leveraging to fulfil the promise of health behaviour. *American Journal of Preventive Medicine*, 22: 320–323.

Tattersall, R. (2002). The expert patient: a new approach to chronic disease management for the twenty-first century. *Journal of the Royal College of Physicians*, 2: 227–229.

Walter, F. M., Emery, J., Braithwaite, D. and Marteua, T. M. (2004). Lay understanding of familial risk of common chronic diseases: a systematic review and synthesis of qualitative research. *Annals of Family Medicine*, 2: 583–594.

Whitlock, E. P., Orleans, T. C., Pender, N. and Allan, J. (2002). Evaluating primary care behavioural counselling interventions: an evidence based approach. *American Journal of Preventive Medicine*, 22: 267–284.

Whitmore, J. (2002). *Coaching for Performance: Growing People, Performance and Purpose*, 3rd edition. London, Nicholas Brealey Publishing.

Wilson, P. M. (2001). A policy analysis of the Expert Patient in the United Kingdom: self care as an expression of pastoral power? *Health & Social Care in the Community*, 9: 134–142.

Yusem, S. H., Rosenberg, K. D., Dixon-Gray, L. and Liu, J. (2004). Public health nursing acceptance of the 5 A's protocol for prenatal smoking cessation. *Californian Journal of Health Promotion*, 2: 1–10.

Resources

The website for Aaron Beck founder of Cognitive Therapy: www.beck-institute.com

The Department of Health website: www.dh.gov.uk

The National Institute for Clinical Excellence: website www.nice.co.uk

Skills for Health coving the competencies needed for the National Occupational Standards: www.skillsforhealth.org.uk

Force-field analysis: www.mindtools.com/pages/article/newTED_06.htm

Inner game website: www.theinnergame.com/

All of the following handouts and advice boxes can be found as individual pdfs on the website at www.blackwellpublishing.com/thew

Advice box 1.1 Knowing your policy: national and local

Consider the following questions; if they are difficult to answer, you need to look further into policy drivers and legislation. Good places to begin are the Department of Health website (www.doh.) and the National Institute for Clinical Excellence (www.nice.co.uk).

- What are the current policies influencing your
  Professional discipline?
  Service area?
- When was the last time you updated this? (If 6 months + look again)
- Could you articulate these policies to someone else?
- Besides policy, has there been any legislative changes that impact on your role or service area?
- How do you see these changes and current drivers affecting your practice?

Advice box 1.2 Good case management

Before embarking on a new piece of work with a client consider how this work fits into their care plan.

Communicate your intentions to the case manager if this is not you.
If you are the care/case manager be sure that you are the most appropriate person to undertake this work.
Make sure that your work is appropriately communicated to others in the care team if they are engaged in work that overlaps or may support/benefit yours.
Decide on the most appropriate way to evaluate your effectiveness within care planning.

Advice box 1.3 Practice reflection

The following questions offer a guide for reflection on practice.

Write your answers to the following guiding questions taking the most recent contact with a client:

- What was the purpose of the client contact and did they know this (you cannot guess here, only answer yes if the purpose was explicitly acknowledged)?
- How did you reach agreement on how to proceed?
- How did you explain the reason for the activity you undertook?
- How did you elicit their feedback and view of the contact and activity?
- In view of your answers, did you optimise the effectiveness of this contact?
- What would you change next time?

Advice box 1.4 Analysis of positive and negative forces

Force-field analysis can be worked with like this:

1. What is your current situation?
2. What is the situation you would like?
3. What will happen if you do nothing to change this situation?
4. List all the forces driving you towards your ideal situation.
5. List all the forces restraining you from moving towards your ideal situation.
6. Explore each of the forces: Are they real? Can they be changed? Which are the key restraining forces?
7. Give a score to each of the forces using a number from (1) extremely weak to (10) extremely strong.
8. Chart the forces by listing the driving forces on the left and restraining forces on the right.
9. You can then visualise the forces and decide whether change is possible and how you can address the situation.

Movement towards your ideal situation can be developed by decreasing the power of the restraining forces and increasing the power of the driving forces.

Advice box 1.5 Achieving inner potential

You can improve your performance in any area be it sport, rehabilitation or success in examinations by maximising your inner potential and minimising the obstacles.

Performance = potential minus interference

When working with clients you may consider this life equation.

Identify an area in your life you wish to change.

The outer game: Identify all the obstacles – every single one of them – and find a practical solution to each.

The inner game: Now focus wholeheartedly on working positively to create the solution you seek. Imagine yourself achieving your goal. Use imagery, positive thinking, will power and all the support systems at your disposal.

Advice box 1.6 The GROW model

The GROW model is a forward-moving model which focuses on a journey towards chosen goals.

Goal. Here the client identifies their goal. The chosen goal must be
Clear
Workable
Non-conflicting with other areas of life.
The individual must be motivated to achieve the goal.

Reality. Here the client reviews their current reality in relation to their goal.

The client's needs should be guided to fully consider the realities of their current situation.

Options. The client is encouraged to identify as many options as possible.

Way forward. The client then *commits* to working towards their goal.
All possible obstacles are identified.
A practical plane with time frames is set.
Support systems are agreed.

The health professional works as a guide through the process using questions to encourage and challenge as appropriate.

Advice box 1.7 Problem lists

In an early contact, ask the client to list the problems they are having at present. These may be directly related to their health problems or peripheral problems. Using the problem list ask them the following: What is the greatest problem on the list? Is there a problem on the list that if solved would improve other problems? Is there a problem that if left would result in a crisis?

From the problem list the practitioner can begin to negotiate the best place to start and also understand the priorities from the client's point of view. For example, it may appear that the main problem is the experience of chronic pain when in fact it is the effect of this on intimacy with a partner and lack of meaningful activity. See Handout 1.4 for a problem-solving method.

Handout 1.1 Reviewing your life

Life review activity. Photocopy three copies of this handout and invite the individual to undertake a 'life review' using the pyramid template.

Life review exercise. Take three copies of this pyramid. Take some time to reflect on and review your life so far.

1. In Pyramid A: identify how satisfied are you in these areas of your life so far.
2. In Pyramid B: identify what you would like to be happening in these areas in the future to increase your well-being.
3. In Pyramid C: identify some steps you can take in any of these areas to increase your happiness and well-being.

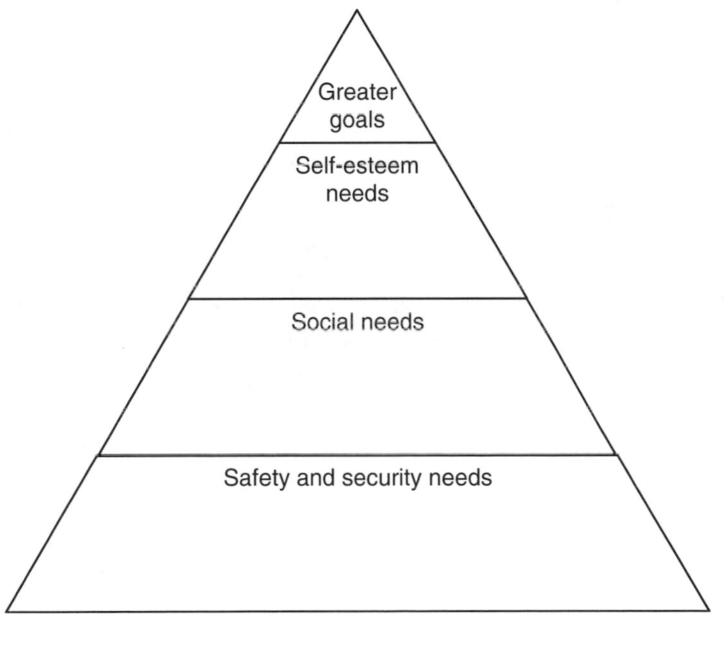

Handout 1.2 Achieving change and goals

The GROW model is a forward-moving model which has been used in sport, business and life coaching to help people make life changes.

Goal. Identify your goal. It must be clear, workable and should not conflict with other priorities you have. Choose a goal you really want to achieve and that means something positive for you.

Reality. What is your situation now in relation to your goal? What are the obstacles and what factors are in your favour.

Options. Identify as many as possible options as you can to choose to help you choose your goal.

Way forward. Now *commit* to achieve your goal. Identify and plan solutions for all the obstacles. Make a practical plan with time frames. What support systems do you need? Put everything in place and get started. Make a date when you will review your progress.

Handout 1.3 The strengths model case management (based on the concept described in Morgan, 1996)

Using the table below, apply the three questions across the top to the areas in the left column. You can start anywhere on the table and change the areas to better represent your areas of practice. Try and avoid problem-solving hopes for the future at this point: the aim is to engage aspirations however unrealistic it may sound at this point, and then plan to get as near as possible to them as goals.

You can look at how the preferences and strategies which worked in the past can apply now. This enables you to engage the client in coping-strategy enhancement, and you can therefore develop current and historical coping as well as teaching new strategies.

Where clients do not know what to put in the 'future' boxes you can see the intervention being one where you explore and find out. Equally, some clients may wish the future to be a continuation of the current or may wish to return to the past state, which are both worthy of attention.

	What has worked for me in the past?	**What is my current situation?**	**What do I want for the future?**
Health			
Occupation			
Leisure			
Accommodation			
Social network			
Managing at home			
Other			

Handout 1.4 Six step problem solving (adapted from Free, 2007)

This can be undertaken with individuals and with a group or family. You are aiming to have two outcomes: to educate the client on a problem-solving method and to work on a problem. Take each step in turn and follow the instructions given below.

1. *Problem definition*: This is an important step to get right. You will need to develop a succinct statement of the problem, saying what the problem is and how it affects the client/family. You can also have some discussion about what would change if this problem was solved. When working with groups you may work on one member's problem and elicit contributions from the other members. When applied with a family, work on a problem for the whole family, starting with something manageable, making sure this is not attributed to a single person.

2. *Possible solutions*: List all the possible solutions without deciding their merits at this point. In groups/family try and have at least one contribution from each participant.

3. *Pros and cons*: Take each solution in turn, weigh its benefits and pitfalls, and give an indication on how best it fits the problem.

4. *Choose a solution*: Choose one of the solutions from above, based on which one came out as being the best fit. Sometimes, this will be a hybrid of more than one solution.

5. *Plan*: Make a plan with the person(s) implementing the solution on who will do it, where, when and how.

6. *Review*: This stage follows the above at a later specified date as you end stage 5. You are reviewing both the success of the strategy and the use of this problem-solving method. Where the problem has not been resolved you would then review the problem definition and repeat the method.

You can use the following worksheet with your client.

Problem-solving worksheet

1. Problem definition: The problem is … which stops me/affects me by … and I feel … when this happens.
   If I solved this problem I would.

2. Possible solutions:

3. Pros and cons:

Pros

Cons

Pros

Cons

Pros

Cons

Pros

Cons

Pros

Cons

Pros

Cons

4. Choose a solution (or blend more than one).

5. Make a plan: think who, what, when, where and how.

6. (a) Date of review:

   (b) Review and revise the plan:

2. *Food and Lifestyle: Healthy Eating and Weight Management*

Pinki Sahota

Introduction

A healthy well-balanced diet is linked to maintaining health and reducing the risk of developing many common diseases such as heart disease, hypertension, Type 2 diabetes, stroke and certain cancers (DH, 1994; WHO, 2003). Obesity is recognised as a risk factor in the development of many of these diseases and consequently its increasing prevalence has been acknowledged as a major concern for public health (Byers and Sedjo 2007). The treatment and prevention of obesity has therefore been prioritised within public health policy (DH, 2004b) and the important role of primary care acknowledged.

The primary health care team has an important role in the identification, assessment and management of overweight and obese adults. A 'typical' National Health Service (NHS) general practice with a list size of 6000 will have approximately 1000 adults who are obese (body mass index [BMI] ≥ 30 kg/m^2) and 50 adults who have severe obesity (BMI ≥ 40 kg/m^2) (DH, 2005; Royal College of General Practitioners, 2005). Furthermore, the Department of Health (DH) has stated that primary care should 'use every opportunity to promote healthy lifestyles' and should provide advice on diet, weight reduction and exercise (National Audit Office, 2001).

Many weight-loss programmes for adults are based on dietary, exercise and behavioural components. Individually each of these components tends to be of limited effectiveness in terms of short- and long-term weight loss (Curioni and Lourenco, 2005; Dansinger *et al.*, 2005; Tsai and Wadden, 2005). However, when these approaches are combined – for example, dietary modification and behavioural therapy – effectiveness is increased compared to diet alone (Glenny *et al.*, 1997).

This chapter will focus on the approach that promotes dietary change based on current healthy eating guidelines with low calorie intake combined with behavioural modification for the treatment of obesity. The advice is based on the recent Department of Health Care Pathway (DH, 2006) and the National Institute for Clinical Excellence (NICE) guidelines for obesity (NICE, 2006). The prevalence, causes and health risks of obesity including the benefits of weight loss will be discussed in order to provide the practitioner with the justification and evidence to help promote behaviour change in their clients. The principles of weight management will be outlined including assessment, safe and realistic weight loss, monitoring and weight maintenance. Behaviour change strategies supported by handouts offering practical suggestions to encourage dietary changes are provided.

Prevalence

The prevalence of overweight and obesity in adults in England has trebled during the past 25 years (see Table 2.1).

The National Audit Office (NAO, 2001) identified that obesity is more prevalent with increasing age in both men and women; being about three times greater in people aged 55–64 years than in people aged 16–24 years. It is also prevalent among people with low educational attainment, low income or manual occupations, and in those living in Scotland and Wales compared with England. There are gender differences with women being more likely to be obese than men, particularly in people from Indian, Pakistani or black Caribbean descent (DH, 2004a).

Causes

Less than 1 in 100 obese people have a 'medical' cause. Conditions such as Cushing's disease and an underactive thyroid are rare

Table 2.1 The percentage of adult men and women who are obese in England as demonstrated in various surveys over 25 years (DH, 2004a).

	1980	1986–1987	1991–1992	1993	1997	2000	2004
Men							
Obese (BMI > 30)	6	7	12	13	17	21	24
Women							
Obese (BMI > 30)	8	12	16	16	20	23	24

causes of weight gain. In addition, some medicines such as steroids, some antidepressants, sulphonylureas and sodium valproate may contribute to weight gain.

Obesity tends to run in families; however, genetics cannot only be responsible for the current obesity epidemic. It is widely accepted that obesity is caused by the interaction between genetics and environmental factors and although the genetics cannot be altered, it is possible to modify environmental factors and thereby influence the development of obesity.

Environmental factors consist of a number of social, psychological and behavioural factors and include:

- *Inactivity.* Reduced physical activity and increased eating behaviour.
- *Diet and eating habits leading to increased food and drink intake.* An increase in weight can result from as little as 50–60 calories a day in excess and/or reduced physical activity, the consequence of which is over 2.4 kg increase in weight by the end of one year (House of Commons Health Select Committee 2004; WHO, 2006). The tendency for weight gain to occur over years for many people means that it is often unnoticed until a person is already overweight or obese and showing signs of associated co-morbidities.
- *Heavy drinking.*
- *Smoking cessation.* Up to 80% of people who quit smoking gain weight and fear of this is a major barrier to smoking cessation.
- *Lower educational attainment, low socioeconomic status, poverty and living in deprived urban areas.* Many surveys suggest that there is a strong correlation between obesity and social deprivation (Rennie and Jebb, 2005).
- *Depression, anxiety and eating disorders.* For example, binge-eating disorder and night eating syndrome are associated with obesity.

Health risks of obesity

The risk of developing health problems increases steadily from a body mass index (BMI) of 25–30 kg/m^2 and increases more rapidly at higher BMI's (Table 2.2). For example,

- The risk of developing diabetes is 40 times greater if the BMI is greater than 35 kg/m^2

Table 2.2 Health risks associated with overweight and obesity in adults.

Greatly increased risk (relative risk > 3)	Moderately increased risk (relative risk 2–3)	Slightly increased risk (relative risk 1–2)
Type 2 diabetes	Coronary heart disease	Cancer (breast in postmenopausal women, endometrium, colon)
Gall bladder diseases	Hypertension	Reproductive hormone abnormalities
Dyslipidaemia	Osteoarthritis (knees and hips)	Polycystic ovary syndrome
Metabolic syndrome	Hyperuricaemia and gout	Impaired fertility
Breathlessness		Low back pain
Sleep apnoea		Increased risk of anaesthetic complications
		Fetal defects associated with maternal obesity

- The risk of coronary heart disease is doubled if the BMI is greater than 25 kg/m^2 and nearly quadrupled if it is 29 kg/m^2 or more.

Health risk and site of excess body fat – apples and pears

In addition to the health risks associated with excess body fat, the site of the excess fat is also linked to health risks. The 'android' pattern of excess central intra-abdominal fat (apple-shape), characteristic of obese men, is associated with hypertension, hyperlipidaemia, glucose intolerance and cardiovascular disease. This is also called the insulin-resistance syndrome, the central obesity syndrome, the metabolic syndrome or syndrome X. In contrast, the 'gynoid' pattern of excess subcutaneous fat distributed about the hips and thighs (pear-shape) is more characteristic of women and is less strongly associated with these problems. In addition to the physical problems, the psychological and social burdens of obesity can be significant: social stigma, low self-esteem, reduced mobility and a generally poorer quality of life are common experiences for many obese people.

What are the benefits of losing weight?

Weight loss in overweight and obese people has been shown to produce a variety of health benefits. Even a moderate weight loss of 5–10% can result in substantial health gains (Jebb, 2004).

Table 2.3 Benefits of 10% weight loss.

Condition	Health benefit
Mortality	20–25% fall in overall mortality
	30–40% fall in diabetes-related deaths
	40–50% fall in obesity-related cancer deaths
Blood pressure	10 mm Hg fall in diastolic and systolic pressures
Diabetes	Up to a 50% fall in fasting blood glucose
	More than a 50% reduction in risk of developing diabetes
Lipids	Fall of 10% total cholesterol, 15% low-density lipoprotein (LDL) cholesterol and 30% triglycerides
	Increase of 8% high-density lipoprotein (HDL) cholesterol

A 10 kg weight loss in a person with an initial weight of 100 kg with co-morbidities would be expected to have the benefits (Table 2.3).

Assessment

The aim of the first appointment should be assessment only. This should include establishing a rapport with the client and to increase the practitioner's level of understanding of the client's weight history including previous weight-loss attempts, any barriers and level of motivation. It is important at this stage to ensure that the patient feels understood and considers himself as an equal partner in planning a way forward.

Body mass index

Overweight or obesity can be assessed by measuring a patient's BMI.

To calculate a patient's BMI, divide their weight in kilograms by the square of their height in metres.

> So, for example, if for someone who weighs 70 kg and is 1.75 metres tall, their BMI is 70/1.75 × 1.75, which is 22.9.

All patients should have their BMI recorded because there is strong evidence for a link between the increasing prevalence of co-morbidities and increasing BMI (Table 2.4).

People should be considered for intervention if their BMI is 30 or more, or if it is 28 or more with co-morbidities.

Table 2.4 Classification of BMI.

Classification	BMI	Risk of co-morbidities
Underweight	<18.5	Low (but increased risk of other clinical problems)
Desirable weight	18.5–24.9	Average
Overweight	25.0–29.9	Mildly increased
Obese	>30.0	
Class I	30.0–34.9	Moderate
Class II	35.0–39.9	High
Class III	>40.0	Markedly increased
(severely or morbidly obese)		

A few points to be aware of when interpreting BMI

- Increasing weight carries a higher risk for Asian populations, who are known to suffer greater health problems at a lower BMI.
- The cut-off BMI level for observed risk in overweight varies from 22 to 25 in different Asian populations. For high risk, it varies from 26 to 31.
- People who are physically very active have greater proportions of lean tissue. Depending on the level of activity, these people will have a high BMI and therefore BMI can be a less accurate predictor of risk.
- Other people for whom BMI may not be an accurate reflection of weight status include those who are older, very short or very tall.

The best way to assess obesity and associated health risks is to use a combination of BMI, waist circumference and body shape.

Waist circumference
The client's waist circumference should be measured according to the World Health Organization (WHO) guidelines, which recommend using the midpoint between the lowest rib and the top of the right iliac crest.

	Healthy waist	Risk to health
Men	Up to 40″ (102 cm)	40″ (102 cm) or more
Women	Up to 35″ (88 cm)	35″ (88 cm) or more
Asian men		≥ 90 cm
Asian women		≥ 80 cm

Risks to health from a high waist circumference include increased visceral fat mass and co-morbidities, including metabolic syndrome.

Once the patient's BMI and waist circumference have been measured it is suggested that other information be considered. The following information is provided as a guide and specific information will vary from individual to individual.

- *Medical risk factors*: Hypertension, hyperlipidaemia, impaired glucose tolerance.
- *Medical history*: For example, diabetes, coronary heart disease, respiratory disease, osteoarthritis.
- *Lifelong weight and dieting history*: To identify previous experiences of weight reduction and patterns of weight-cycling.
- *Family weight history*: To identify possible genetic factors.
- *Eating behaviour history*: To identify disordered eating, for example, binge-eating disorder.
- *Dietary history*: Assess current food and drink intake.

It is helpful to know about your client's eating habits; what, when and how much they currently eat and how they feel when they eat, for example, hungry, upset, bored.

An estimate of usual food intake or their diet in the previous 24 hours is often inaccurate and therefore it is suggested that a self-monitoring 3-day or 7-day diary may help clients to track their food intake and their feelings about their weight (Handout 2.1).

Under-reporting

Although a detailed diary of food and drink that they consume over an average week is helpful and can form the basis for discussing dietary change, it must be noted that overweight or obese client tend to under-report their food intake (Lara *et al.*, 2004). If this is suspected, then careful questioning about food intake is useful (see Advice box 2.1).

Understanding the process of change

The Stages of Change Transtheoretical model developed by Prochaska and Diclemente (1982) is a useful model that can be applied to assess the level of motivation and the stage of change of the client. The model is designed to assess readiness to change and level of motivation of the client and guide the practitioner to provide appropriate support to facilitate the behaviour change process. The type of support appropriate for each stage of change is summarised in Table 2.5.

Table 2.5 Use of the stages of change model to promote weight control among clients.

Stages of change	Process of change	Primary care practitioner
Pre-contemplation	Consciousness-raising	Discuss with the client any problems associated with being overweight and the feasibility of weight loss
Contemplation	Recognition of the benefits of change	Discuss with the client the potential benefits to them of proposed change
Determination or preparation	Identification of barriers	Assist client in identifying potential barriers they may face and how these can be addressed and emphasise the relative benefits
Action	Programme of change	Work with the client to work out a plan for weight loss and identify support mechanisms
Maintenance	Follow-up and continuing support	Organise routine follow-up and discuss with client the likelihood of relapse

Obesity management in primary care

The priority in weight management should be to reduce risk factors for the clients. Very small degrees of weight loss produce health benefits, but significant changes result after a loss of 5–10%. For some individuals, a weight loss of as little as 7–12 lb (3.0–5.5 kg) can achieve health benefits.

Table 2.6 indicates what a 5% or 10% weight loss would mean in actual weight.

Management

The aim of management is to help people to (see Advice box 2.2)

- Regularise eating behaviour.
- Promote healthy eating with a focus on reducing energy or calorie intake.

Table 2.6 What a weight loss of 5% and 10% means in terms of actual weight.

Starting weight	5% means losing	10% means losing
11 stone (70 kg)	8 lb (3.5 kg)	1 stone 2 lb (7 kg)
14 stone (89 kg)	10 lb (4.5 kg)	1 stone 6 lb (9 kg)
16 stone (102 kg)	11 lb (5 kg)	1 stone 8 lb (10 kg)
18 stone (115 kg)	13 lb (6 kg)	1 stone 11 lb (11.5 kg)
20 stone (127 kg)	1 stone (6.5 kg)	2 stone (13 kg)

- Increase self-awareness about day-to-day behaviours that affect intake and planning coping strategies to prevent relapses.

Regularise eating behaviour

The assessment using the diary (Handout 2.1) may have indicated an erratic eating pattern such as skipping meals, restrained eating followed by compensatory overeating, frequent snacking or binge-eating. Snacking has been found to correlate with a higher BMI in adults aged between 20 and 59 years (Howarth *et al.*, 2007). Discussion about previous attempts of weight reducing may have indicated a pattern of 'weight-cycling'. The aim is to stabilise eating behaviour and weight prior to any attempt to reduce weight.

1. Aim to eat three meals and two snacks. In an attempt to avoid constant snacking or 'grazing' behaviour the individual should be encouraged to eat three meals and two snacks per day so as so avoid long periods without food. It is important to include breakfast as research has shown that the diets of those who miss breakfast are higher in fat and consequently higher in calories.
2. Include two snacks per day. Long periods without food often lead to hunger and snacking or picking. Snack foods such as confectionary, cake and biscuits are often high in fat and/or sugar. Therefore, patients should be encouraged to plan ahead by including snacks such as fruit, raw vegetables and sugar-free drinks at times when they feel they are most vulnerable to making inappropriate choices. Evenings are a common time for overeating through snacking or drinking alcohol. Strategies such as pre-prepared raw vegetables or fruits in the fridge may be helpful.

To regularise eating behaviour the following need to be considered in advance:

- When to eat
- What to eat
- How much to eat.

Advantages of regular eating

- It provides the body with adequate nutrition and thus reduces strong craving for foods that are going to set off overeating.
- It permits eating only at certain times and makes it clear when not to eat.
- It is better to eat regularly than to depend on distorted body signals.
- It reduces tendencies to delay eating.

It is important to eat according to the planned pattern of regular eating and not by sensation of hunger and other urges to eat. Overeating and dieting disrupts the normal mechanisms that control sensation of hunger and fullness. Therefore, these sensations should not be trusted at this early stage. The normal sensations of hunger and fullness will gradually return with eating regularly (without overeating and dieting). Patients should be advised to consider the following when planning their diet:

- Ensure that there is no gap longer than four hours between planned meals and snacks.
- Make every effort to stick to the meal plan and review progress at the end of each day.
- Do not skip meals or snacks, as this will make them vulnerable to overeating.
- Avoid eating in between planned meals and snacks.
- Avoid eating anything that is known to trigger overeating.
- Plan in advance what is to be eaten – deciding what to eat can be a problem when hungry.
- Ensure an average sized portion at every meal. This can be determined by
    - Looking at the information on non-diet food packages.
    - Looking at handout on portion sizes.
- Write down a meal plan for meals each day to cut down the worry about what to have.

If patients find it a struggle to change their eating habits all at once, introduce regular eating in stages. For example, plan breakfast every day for a week, breakfast and lunch every day for the second week.

Diet and weight reduction

With specific reference to the prevention of obesity, WHO concluded in 2003 that 'there is convincing evidence that a high intake of energy dense foods promotes weight gain' and that 'the majority of studies show that a high intake of Non-starch Polysaccharide (NSP) (dietary fibre) promotes weight loss'. The report highlighted that 'energy dense foods tend to be high in fat (e.g. butter, oils, fried foods), sugars or starch while lower-energy foods have a high fibre and water content (e.g. fruit and vegetables, whole grain cereals)'. The report also concluded that there was 'probable' evidence on increased consumption of sweetened drinks and large portion sizes increasing risk of weight gain and obesity. This combined with the fact that most people in the UK eat less than three items of fruit and vegetables a day (DH, 2002) describes a diet that is lacking in nutrition as well as being high in fat and sugar.

Healthy eating

Although it is accepted that any diet that reduces calorie intake can lead to weight loss, it is important that a sensible approach is taken. Diets aimed at promoting weight loss should be in line with general healthy eating guidelines and additionally should be:

- Acceptable to the person
- Nutritionally sound
- Sustainable in the long term.

Ideally, dietary recommendations should be extended to the family, particularly where more than one member is obese. This can help in motivational factors and also in gaining support for the healthy eating ethos.

Promoting dietary change (Handouts 2.2 and 2.6)

The following factors should be considered when offering advice on dietary modification:

- Practical – based on everyday foods rather than special dietary products, or expensive and inaccessible foods.
- Positive – stress what can be eaten rather than what should be avoided.

- Personalised – tailored to individual needs (age, sex, weight and activity levels).
- Palatable – include foods liked.
- Possible – take into account personal factors (income, cooking skills, work patterns, family, etc.).

Standard UK population recommendations on 'healthy eating' are based on the recommendations of the Committee on the Medical Aspects of Food Policy (COMA) (National Audit Office, 2001; DH, 2005; Royal College of General Practitioners, 2005) and subsequently the Scientific Advisory Committee on Nutrition (SACN 2003) (DH, 2006). This advice is reflected in the 'National food guide, the Eatwell Plate' (FSA, 2007). See Figure 2.1.

The main messages that are promoted by this model are of variety, balance and moderation. The diet includes a variety of foods from all the food groups, and there are no 'good or bad' foods. This understanding is fundamental and underpins the core healthy eating principles which aim to engender a healthy attitude towards food and eating that can be sustained in the long term.

The model encourages messages of balance and moderation through the consumption of foods from the five food groups in the proportions reflected. It promotes a diet that is nutritionally sound

The eatwell plate
FOOD STANDARDS AGENCY
food.gov.uk
Use the eatwell plate to help you get the balance right. It shows how much of what you eat should come from each food group.
Fruit and vegetables
Bread, rice, potatoes, pasta and other starchy foods
Meat, fish, eggs, beans and other non-dairy sources of protein
Foods and drinks high in fat and/or sugar
Milk and dairy foods

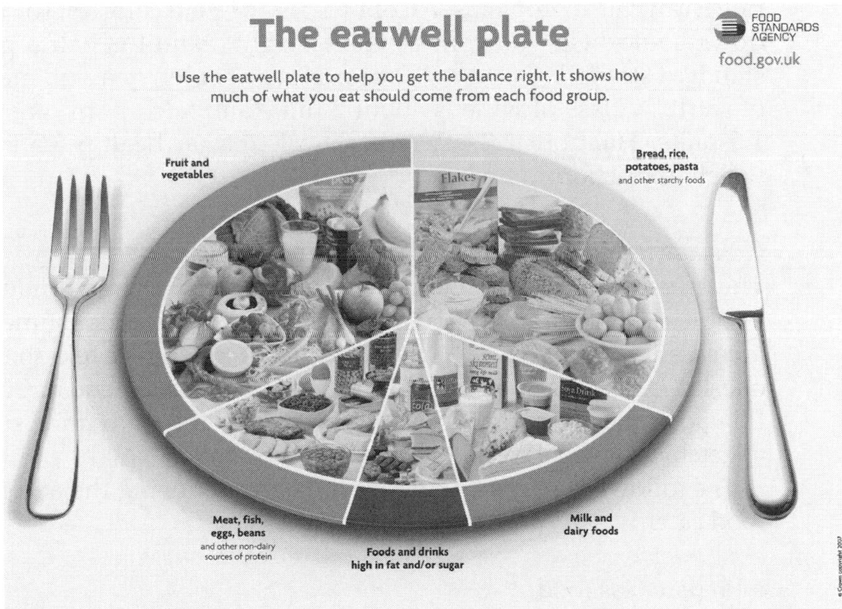

Fig. 2.1 The Eatwell Plate.

through encouraging the consumption of a variety of foods from all the five food groups, thereby encouraging adequate intake of nutrients to maintain health.

The main messages are to:

- Eat five or more portions of a range of fruit and vegetables per day.
- Base meals on starchy foods such as wholemeal bread, pasta, rice, cereal, potatoes or other root vegetables.
- Reduce intake of foods high in fat and sugar.
- Use cooking methods that reduce fat, for example, grilling and steaming, and limit the addition of fat in cooking.
- Avoid drinks high in sugar; drink sugar-free drinks or water.
- Reduce alcohol intake as alcohol is high in calories.
- Consume fewer snacks high in fat or sugar – snack on fruits and vegetables instead.

Alcohol

Regarding alcohol intake, the DH advises that men should not drink more than 3–4 units of alcohol per day, and women should drink no more than 2–3 units of alcohol per day. These daily benchmarks apply whether individuals drink every day, once or twice a week, or occasionally. The FSA also advises consumers that 'There is nothing wrong with having the occasional drink. But drinking too much can cause problems. Alcohol is also high in calories, so cutting down could help you control your weight. A unit is half a pint of standard strength (3–5% ABV) beer, lager or cider, or a pub measure of spirit. A glass of wine is about 2 units and 'alco-pops' are about 1.5 units. Handout 2.2 offers practical tips on healthy eating for weight reduction.

How much to eat: Portion sizes

The assessment using the diary (Handouts 2.4 and 2.5) may have indicated that large portions of food maybe being consumed. As increased portion sizes have been linked to the development of obesity it is recommended that patients should be encouraged to fill upon foods that have low energy density and high fibre, such as vegetables or salad, or higher-fibre starchy foods.

The following practical tips are aimed at reducing the amount of food eaten:

- Prepare less food
- Begin to select smaller helpings
- Eat from a smaller plate

- Never buy large or super-size portions
- Eat more slowly
- Stop eating when you no longer feel hungry, rather than waiting until you feel full.

Handout 2.6 indicates appropriate portion sizes to include in the diet.

Other diets

Some individuals may choose to attend commercial organisations for additional advice and support. This should complement the practice approach. Low-calorie diets (1000–1500 kcal/day) are proven effective methods of weight loss. Very-low-calorie diets (VLCDs) should only be used under medical supervision and ideally with input from a registered dietitian. Fad diets or highly restrictive diets such as low-carbohydrate, high-protein diets should be avoided; they are likely to be unsustainable and their long-term impact on health remains unclear. Special diets which are often advertised are not usually helpful (Dansinger *et al.*, 2005). This is because after losing weight, if old eating habits remain, the weight often goes straight back on. It is usually not a special diet that is needed, but changing to a normal healthy balanced diet – for good.

Behavioural change/modification

Behaviour modification therapy is based on the assumption that eating behaviour is acquired and maintained through the immediate environment but can be relearned if the environment is manipulated.

Often people eat in response to cues not particularly associated with hunger. Cues such as emotional, social or associated with a particular time or place are responsible for initiating eating. Behavioural modification aims to help individuals to recognise these cues and then develop strategies to avoid or change these cues in order to establish a healthier eating pattern (Shaw *et al.*, 2005). The practical principles of behaviour modification to aid weight loss are summarised in Handout 2.7. However maintaining weight loss in the chronically obese even after intensive lifestyle intervention can often be of short term benefit (Bruun *et al.*, 2007) and relapse to previous eating habits is common. There is a general stigma attached to being obese particularly in younger adults, where sexual attraction is rated as less desirable in a potential partner over and above disability (Chen and Brown, 2005). It is therefore inevitable that as a person loses weight, there may be some increase in libido, but there may also be some disquiet expressed by the partners as new found sexual confidence grows and the 'usual' relationship starts to unfold.

Finally, it must be acknowledged that treatment of obesity can feel a thankless task as relapse is common. However, if relapse is viewed not as a failure but as a stepping stone to future change, then both you and your client will be less easily discouraged. Handout 2.3 gives suggestions on helping your patients dealing with relapse.

Remember, change takes time and therefore realistic expectations should be discussed at the outset. Most importantly stay positive – if this idea does not work, remember that another one might.

Conclusion

This chapter has suggested a practical and safe approach to weight management. There is no compensating for the motivated individual in terms of successful weight loss. There is now worldwide concerted effort to reduce the health burden created by poor diets and sedentary lives. It is costing the world millions in health care utility but also in loss of life years. The problem is not confined to the UK or westernised cultures, there are worrying trends emerging for the developing countries.

Health care professionals are ideally suited to support weight loss programmes with individuals they see within their main care. The benefits of a healthy balanced diet are not confined to being the 'ideal' weight but consuming a healthy diet will contribute to reducing the risk of developing conditions associated with obesity such as heart disease, hypertension, Type 2 diabetes, stroke and certain cancers. If long-lasting weight loss is to be achieved, diets need to be underpinned by behavioural change, and motivational strategies which include planned coping mechanisms for clients so that success is maximised.

Generally, many problems of lifestyle could be attributed to lifestyle behaviours that include eating and drinking. Although weight management maybe perceived as common sense, it can be a challenging and lengthy process; however, the benefits can be life changing as well as life saving.

References

Byers, T. and Sedjo, R. L. (2007). Public health response to the obesity epidemic: too soon or too late? *Journal of Nutrition*, 137(2): 488–492.

Bruun, J. M., Madsen, E. L. and Richelsen, B. (2007). Weight loss maintenance in severely obese adults after an intensive lifestyle intervention: 2- to 4-year follow-up. *Obesity*, 15: 413–420.

Curioni, C. C. and Lourenço, P. M. (2005). Long-term weight loss after diet and exercise: a systematic review. *International Journal of Obesity*, 29(10): 1168–1174.

Dansinger, M. L., Gleasonm, J. A., Griffithm, J. L., Selkerm, H. P. and Schaeferm, E. J. (2005). Comparison of the Atkins, Ornish, Weight Watchers, and Zone diets for weight loss and heart disease risk reduction: a randomized trial. *Journal of the American Medical Association*, 293: 43–53.

DH (1991). *Dietary Reference Values for Food Energy and Nutrients for the United Kingdom. Report of the Panel on Dietary Reference Values of the Committee on Medical Aspects of Food Policy*. London, HMSO.

DH (1994). *Nutritional Aspects of Cardiovascular Disease*. London, HMSO.

DH (1998). *Nutritional Aspects of the Development of Cancer. Report of the Working Group on Diet and Cancer of the Committee on Medical Aspects of Food and Nutrition Policy*. London, The Stationery Office.

DH (2002). *The National Diet and Nutrition Survey*. London, HMSO.

DH (2004a). *Health Survey for England*. http://www.dh.gov.uk/PublicationsAndStatistics/PublishedSurvey/HealthSurveyForEngland. Accessed April 2007.

DH (2004b). *'Choosing Health': Making Healthy Choices Easier*. London, The Stationery Office. Accessed June 2006.

DH (2005). *Health Survey for England – Trends*. London, Department of Health.

DH (2006). Obesity care pathway and your weight, your health. *Department of Health Central Office of Information* www.dh.gov.uk/en/Publicationsandstatistics/Publications/PublicationsPolicyAndGuidance/DH_4134408. Accessed June 2006.

FSA (2007). The Eatwell Plate. http://www.eatwell.gov.uk/healthydiet/eatwellplate/. Food Standards Agency.

Glenny, A., O'Meara, S., Melville, A., Sheldon, T. A. and Wilson, C. (1997). Systematic review of interventions for the prevention and treatment of obesity and the maintenance of weight loss. *International Journal of Obesity and Related Metabolic Disorders*, 221(9): 715–737.

House of Commons Health Select Committee (2004). *Obesity: Third Report of Session 2003–04*. London, The Stationery Office.

Howarth, N. C., Huang, T. T. K., Roberts, S. B., Lin, H. and McCory, M. A. (2007). Eating patterns and dietary composition in relation to BMI in younger and older adults. *International Journal of Obesity*, 31: 675–684.

Jebb, S. (2004). Obesity: causes and consequences. *Women's Health Medicine*, 1(1): 38–41.

Lara, J. J., Scott, J. A. and Lean, M. E. J. (2004). Intentional mis-reporting of food consumption and its relationship with body mass index and psychological scores in women. *Journal of Human Nutrition and Dietetics*, 17(3): 209–218.

National Audit Office (2001). *Tackling Obesity in England*. London, The Stationery Office.

NICE (2006). *Obesity: The Prevention, Identification, Assessment and Management of Overweight and Obesity in Adults and Children*. Clinical guideline. http://guidance.nice.org.uk/ CG43. Accessed April 2007.

Prochaska, J. O. and DiClemente, C. (1982). *Transtheoretical Approaches: Crossing Traditional Foundations of Therapy*. Homewood, IL, Dow-Jones/Irwin.

Rennie, K. L. and Jebb, S. A. (2005). National prevalence of obesity. Prevalence of obesity in Great Britain. *Obesity Reviews*, 6: 11–12.

Royal College of General Practitioners (2005). Key statistics from general practice. www.rcgp.org.uk/information/publications/information/PDFFact/05SEP05.pdf. Accessed March 2006.

SACN (2003). *Salt and Health*. London, The Stationery Office.

Shaw, K., O'Rourke, P., Del Mar, C. and Kenardy, J. (2005). Psychological interventions for overweight or obesity. *Cochrane Database of Systematic Reviews*, 18(2).

Tsai, A. G. and Wadden, T. A. (2005). Systematic review: an evaluation of major commercial weight loss programs in the United States. *Annals of Internal Medicine*, 142(1): 56–66.

WHO (2003). *Diet, Nutrition and the Prevention of Chronic Disease*. Technical Report Series 916. Geneva, World Health Organization.

WHO (2006). *Obesity: Preventing and Managing the Global Epidemic*. Geneva, World Health Organization.

Key obesity-related websites

- American Dietetic Association: www.eatright.org
- Association for the Study of Obesity (UK): www.aso.org.uk
- British Dietetic Association www.bda.uk.com
- Counterweight Project: www.counterweight.org
- DOM-UK Dietitians in Obesity Management: www.domuk.org/
- Diogenes Project: www.diogenes-eu.org/
- Health Education Board for Scotland: www.hebs.scot.nhs.uk/learningcentre/weightmanagement/index.cfm
- International Association for the Study of Obesity: www.iaso.org
- International Obesity Taskforce Network: www.iotf.org/
- Medscape Weight Management Resource Centre: www.medscape.com/pages/editorial/resourcecenters/public/weightmgmt/rc-weightmgmt.ov
- National Obesity Forum: www.nationalobesityforum.org.uk
- National Institutes of Health, National Heart, Lung and Blood Institute. Clinical guidelines on the identification, evaluation and treatment of overweight and obesity in adults: the evidence report, 1998: www.nhlbi.nih.gov/guidelines/obesity/ob_home.htm

- National Weight Control Registry (USA): www.uchsc.edu/nutrition/WyattJortberg/nwcr.htm
- Scottish Intercollegiate Network: www.sign.ac.uk
- Shape Up America: www.shapeup.org
- Weight Concern: www.weightconcern.com

All of the following handouts and advice boxes can be found as individual pdfs on the website at www.blackwellpublishing.com/thew

Advice box 2.1 Practical tips on healthy eating for weight reduction

Often people tend to underestimate how much they eat, and are apt to believe that their weight problem is out of their personal locus of control. Therefore, there should be some rapport gained at the first assessment session, with careful and sensitive handling regarding the amount and type of food consumed and the levels of exercise engaged in to counteract the calorie intake.

Questions to ask regarding food intake. The following questions maybe helpful in establishing accurate information about food intake and eating habits:

- Do you ever eat biscuits with your tea or coffee?
- Would you ever eat chocolate, cake, pastries?
- How many times a week do you go out in the evenings?
- What sorts of drinks do you have when you go out in the evening?

Factors influencing food intake. Identify social or cultural factors affecting food choice and consequent impact on personal eating habits

Readiness to change (use in association with Handouts 2.1 and 2.2). There is evidence that overweight people are more motivated to lose weight if advised to do so by a health professional. An excellent starting point is a collaborative discussion between the practitioner and client to:

- Explore how the person feels about their weight.
- Understand whether they feel that there are successful solutions.
- Understand their level of awareness of the risks associated with carrying excess weight.

It is important during the assessment stage to establish whether making changes to lose weight is right for this person at this specific time of their life. Changing personal circumstances may have an impact on whether a patient will be able to make changes within their life at a specific time. The following questions can help assess the patient's readiness to change:

- How important is losing weight at the moment?
- What would have to change in your life for you to be able to tackle your weight?
- Are you concerned about your weight?
- Do you believe that you could lose weight?
- How important is it for you to lose weight at the moment?
- Is your weight affecting your life in any way at the moment?
- Do you know that it could really help your blood pressure if you managed to lose a little weight?

If a patient does not appear to be ready to change, try to explore reasons why they may not be ready and what might be done to influence this. Where possible, offer the patient the chance to come back at some future point. Some individuals may be – or appear to be – uncertain about readiness to change. In this case, limited discussion about management options may be helpful.

Advice box 2.2 How to support your patient/client to lose weight

- *Be realistic in setting the goal.* Some people aim to get down to an ideal but unrealistic weight and because this target is too low, they may begin to feel frustrated about poor progress, and give up. Therefore, setting a realistic target based on a weight that was attained within the recent past such as pre-pregnancy, might be more achievable. Once achieved a further target weight can be set if appropriate. As stated above, in most cases, most health benefits come from losing the first 5–10% of weight (often about 5–10 kg).
- *Support a gradual weight loss.* A slow and steady weight loss should be the aim. Very restrictive diets may achieve an impressive initial effect, but most of this is due to loss of water from the muscle stores. Such diets cannot be sustained and therefore the weight is regained. If more than a kilogram per week is lost, it is likely to be muscle tissue rather than fat. It is best to lose an average of 0.5–1 kg per week (1–2 lb per week).

The idea is for patients to gradually readjust their eating habits to a healthier pattern so that the weight lost will be sustained. Eating 500–600 fewer calories per day is a realistic way to lose weight and a weight loss of 0.5–1 kg (1–2 lb) per week can be achieved.

500 fewer calories per day = 3500 fewer calories per week.
3500 calories = 0.5 kg of fat.
Therefore, 0.5 kg of body fat is lost per week.

If patients sustain this reduction in calories for up to 3 months it is possible to lose 6–12 kg.

Other general points. The first kilogram is the easiest to lose. This is because water is lost from the body at first as well as fat. It is important to advice people that the initial kilogram or so may seem to fall off rapidly, but then the weight loss usually slows down. It is important to advise people not to be disheartened by minor increases or levelling off in weight for a few days. It is also important to observe the overall

Advice box 2.2 Continued

trend in weight loss over several months. Regular weighing, advice and encouragement should be offered to maintain motivation.

As individuals get closer to a healthier weight, it is found that weight loss usually slows down. This is because less energy is used to move their weight around and if weight loss was to continue at the same rate, energy intake would need to be reduced further. People can often feel demotivated when this occurs and therefore additional support is required at this stage.

Rewarding and getting family and friends on board with weight loss is vital, if those around the patient are undermining any programme to lose weight, the likelihood of relapse is great. The checklist in Handout 2.7, points to rewards being accrued when weight is lost, it may also be worth finding out how others have reacted when they have announced how much weight they have lost already. There may even be some jealousy in family and friends, even in people who have little to lose. There may also be a situation where others in the family may feel 'threatened' by someone starting to feel more confident with weight loss. This may require a more structured counselling approach from a separate counsellor, especially if relationships start to unfold as the weight starts to drop.

Handout 2.1 How to change your eating habits

- Keep a detailed food diary.
  - Record not only what is eaten but when, where and feelings at the time of eating – for example, bored or depressed.
  - Was it a snack or a main meal?
  - Was the food eaten sitting at the table, watching TV or out shopping?
  - Was the food eaten because it was available rather than wasting it?

- Using the diary identify the occasions when food was eaten in the absence of hunger. Then agree activities that could take place to avoid these situations, for example, phone a friend, go for a walk or start a hobby.

- Eat only at mealtimes, preferably sitting at the table. Plan appropriate snacks into the daily meal pattern.

- Eat slowly and enjoy eating.

- Plan meals for the week and make a shopping list, but it is recommended not to go shopping when feeling hungry.

- Avoid cooking more than is needed. Remove dishes after serving to avoid further helpings.

- Apart from fruit and vegetables, do not leave snack food so it is accessible.

Handout 2.2 What to eat/drink and what to avoid

Eat less sugar

- Do not take sugar in tea or coffee or on cereals. Use sweeteners instead if required.
- Choose water, mineral waters or low-calorie drinks instead of squash or fizzy drinks.
- Avoid sugar coated breakfast cereals.
- Cut down on sweets, chocolates, cakes and biscuits – eat fresh fruits or vegetables instead.
- Use fruit tinned in natural juice than in syrup.

Eat more fibre

- Have a high-fibre breakfast cereal, for example, bran flakes, shredded wheat, muesli or porridge.
- Aim for five helpings of fruit and vegetables per day.
- Include peas, beans, lentils in meals.
- Try wholemeal pasta, brown rice, wholemeal bread.

Drink less alcohol

- If you can, avoid alcohol – it is full of calories and no nutrients.
- If you drink alcohol, alternate alcoholic drinks with mineral water or low-calorie drinks.

Eat less fat

- Grill, steam or casserole food.
- Choose lean cuts of meat or trim off the fat.
- Choose lean mince and drain off the fat.
- Avoid eating the skin on chicken.
- Use semi-skimmed or skimmed milk.
- Choose lower-fat cheeses: for example, edam, gouda or cottage cheese instead of cheddar.
- Cut down on crisp-type snacks.
- Avoid oily salad dressings, mayonnaise and salad cream – try lemon juice or vinegar instead.
- Use less butter or margarine – they are both the same calories.
- Try low-fat spreads and other low-fat products. But read the label as they maybe high in sugar.
- Make sure low-fat yoghurts are also low in sugar.
- Do not put butter or margarine on vegetables.
- Use low-fat yoghurt instead of cream.

Handout 2.3 Dealing with relapse

Relapse is part of the behaviour change process. When this occurs offer the patient support and encouragement. Help them to identify the reasons and developing strategies to avoid relapse from occurring.

- Relapse or setback is more likely to happen if the goals have been too ambitious. Relapses do not just happen, there is always a reason. Identify the causes.
- How are they dealing with unpleasant feelings such as upset, anxiety, stress?
- One way to avoid relapse is to ensure that patients are being realistic about themselves and their eating pattern.
- Set a target that can be achieved (it can always make it more difficult later on).
- If the target set does not work, do not consider the patient or allow them to feel a failure, but try to work out why it did not work.
- Help patients to learn to recognise situations when they are most at risk (keep a record) and have a plan for dealing with each situation.
- Learn from setbacks and help patients to understand why it happened and what they can do to stop it.
- Do not just ignore the relapse, try to change the behaviour or situation that acts as a trigger.
- Do not let the odd setback make you so disheartened that you give up completely.
- Remember one setback does not mean you are a total failure.

Handout 2.4 Diary keeping

Monitoring eating. You can monitor your eating by keeping a diary. This involves recording what you eat and drink, your thoughts and feelings. (An example of how to complete the diary is in Handout 2.5a.)

What do I gain from keeping a diary?

- It provides a detailed picture of your eating.
- It helps to monitor and discover the *connections* between overeating and a particular event, mood, thought or behaviour.
- It helps to identify *trigger factors* for overeating.

Instruction for monitoring (see blank Handout 2.5b)

- Column 1 (time) – Record the time when you eat or drink anything.
- Column 2 (description of food or drink) – Write down all the food or drink you consume during the day. Each item should be written down as soon as possible after it has been eaten. Therefore, it is necessary to keep your diary with you all the time. Provide a simple description of what you ate, for example, bread (thick or thin slice), milk (whole, semi-skimmed or skimmed), sausages (normal or low fat), and so on.
- Column 3 (how much) – Describe the portion in household measures, that is, slices, tablespoons, mugs or cups, brands (e.g. Kellogg's cornflakes), type of food (e.g. white bread or wholemeal bread), biscuits (e.g. digestive, club or penguin), and so on.
- Column 4 – Record activities by writing the duration of each activity, for example, walking 20 minutes.
- Columns 5 and 6 – Use these columns to record thoughts, feelings and emotions that have influenced your eating. If you have overeaten, it is important that you try to specify what the circumstances were in which these episodes occurred and what you were feeling and thinking at the time. Record *positive as well as negative* thoughts and feelings.

Handout 2.5a Example (diet diary)

Time	Description of food/ drink	How much	Activity (minutes)	Thoughts	Feelings
8 a.m.	Weetabix	1			
	Milk – semi-skimmed	1 cup		Still feel full from yesterday.	
	Butter – low fat		Walk (20)	Starting my new diet today.	
	Bread – thin slice (white)	2 slices		I must do well.	Tired.
	Tea – black	2 cups		I should have less than 1000 kcal today.	
1 p.m.	Apple	1			Feel stressed.
	Diet coke	1 can			
5 p.m.			Walk (20)		
6 p.m.	Chocolate biscuits (digestives)	4		I am still hungry. I should not eat.	
				Friend cancelled date.	Feel guilty and unhappy.

Handout 2.5a Continued

Time	Description of food/ drink	How much	Activity (minutes)	Thoughts	Feelings
7 p.m.	Bread – thick (white)	4 slices		I have broken my diet again. I might as well carry on eating.	
	Baked beans – large	1 tin			
	Cheese	2 slices			I am angry with everyone.
				I am too fat.	I am hopeless.
8 p.m.	Peanuts	100 g			
	Ham	2 slices			
	Bread – thick (white)	2 slices		Everything keeps going wrong.	
	Chocolate bar large (Mars bar)	1		Start my diet tomorrow.	
10 p.m.	Hot chocolate – low fat	1 mug		In control	Good

Day………………………………………………………… … … … …………..Date……………………………………………….

Handout 2.5b Blank diet diary

Time	Description of food/drink	How much	Activity (minutes)	Thoughts	Feelings

Day...Date..

Handout 2.6 Healthy eating – portion sizes

To allow some variety in planning your meals, you can use this list to exchange foods for one another and be sure that you are eating a balanced diet.

Group one

Bread and cereal foods – six portions per day. Each of the following foods is roughly the same as one large slice of bread

Bread	one large slice or half a roll.
Breakfast cereal	level cereal bowl of flakes/porridge or two Weetaibix or two Shredded Wheat or small bowl of Museli.
Biscuits	two plain biscuits, for example digestives, or one small chocolate biscuit, or one scone or a slice of fruit bread.
Rice and pasta	four to six tablespoons of cooked pasta/rice.
Potato	two tablespoons of mashed potato or one medium size jacket potato.

Try to eat wholemeal, wholegrain, brown or high-fibre variety.
Where possible avoid
Having them fried (e.g. chips)
Adding too much fat (e.g. thick spread on bread)
Adding rich sauces (e.g. cream/cheese on pasta).

Group two

Fruit and vegetables – five or more portions each day (three fruits and two vegetables/salad).

Vegetables	to cover about one third of the plate
Salad	to cover about one third of half of the plate

Eat a wide variety of fruit (fresh, dried, canned in fruit juice) and vegetables (fresh, frozen, canned).
Where possible avoid adding fat or rich sauces to vegetables or adding sugar or syrup to fruits.

Group three

Milk and milk products – one pint milk or equivalent each day. Each of the following is the same as a glass of milk.

Fruit yoghurt	one 5 ounce carton
Cheese	1 ounce (about the size of your thumb)
Cottage cheese	one small carton
Fromage frais	one carton

This group does not include butter and cream. Choose lower-fat versions whenever you can, for example, semi-skimmed or skimmed milk.

Group four

Meat and meat alternative – two portions each day.

Fish	one fillet (6–8 ounces)
Tinned fish	3 ounces
Red meat	3 ounces (about the size of the palm of your hand) cooked
Chicken	3 ounces (about the size of the palm of your hand) cooked
Eggs	two
Beans and pulses	one small tin or three tablespoons

Meat includes bacon and salami and meat products such as sausages, beefburgers and pate. These all are fairly high-fat choices.
Fish includes fresh, frozen, canned, fish fingers and fish cakes.

Choose lower variety whenever you can, for example,
Meat with the fat cut off
Chicken with the skin removed
Fish without batter.

Tofu (made of soya), beans and pulses are good alternative to meat as they are naturally very low in fat.

Group five

Fatty and sugary foods. Eat in moderation and/or in small amount.

What foods included – margarine, low-fat spread, butter, other spreading fats, cooking oils, oily salad dressings or mayonnaise, cream, chocolate, crisps, biscuits, pastries, cake, puddings, ice-cream, rich sauces and fatty gravies, sweet and sugars.

Some foods in this group will be eaten everyday but should be kept to small amounts, for example, margarine, butter, cooking oils.
Some foods in this group are occasional foods, for example, cream, ice-cream.

Handout 2.7 How to change your eating habits

Try some of these suggestions. Tick the things you already do and put a star * against those you would like to try.

1. Eat only in one room; kitchen or dining room. Do not eat in the bedroom or sitting room.
2. Eat in one place in that room and always put the food you are going to eat on a plate.
3. Eat sitting down.
4. Do not watch TV or read whilst eating.
5. Eat slowly; chew food thoroughly, enjoy each mouthful and put down your knife and fork between bites of food if you are eating too quickly.
6. Limit contact with too much food. Avoid preparing extras or second helpings. Serve food from cooking pans at the stove.
7. Make small portions of food look as larger by putting them on a smaller plate.
8. Scrape plates directly into the bin once you have finished eating.
9. Store leftover foods such as bread, butter, cheese after the meal to avoid nibbling.
10. Do not serve high-calorie sauces with meals.
11. Look for ways to change your recipes to make them lower in fat and sugar.
12. Have lots of variety; vary the types of meat, fish, vegetables and fruits chosen so that meals do not become boring.
13. Make your meals as attractive as possible. Use low-calorie garnishes and spices such as celery, peppers and fresh herbs.
14. Eat meals at regular times to avoid getting too hungry.
15. Spend money you save by not buying cakes, biscuits, sweets, crisps or alcohol on other foods such as strawberries, melon and salmon.
16. Do not buy foods that are not suitable for your diet such as sweets, cakes, crisps and biscuits.
17. Shop after meals and not before. Shopping on an empty stomach usually makes people buy more food than they normally would.
18. Always make a shopping list and stick to it.
19. Plan your day to avoid boredom. Have an interesting activity readily available such as reading, walking, painting or gardening.
20. Reward yourself with things other than food such as an outing, new clothes, make-up, CD, book or magazine.

3. *Getting the Balance Right: Managing Work–Home Conflict*

Jim McKenna and Miranda Thew

Most working age adults spend the majority of their waking lives within the workplace; it is the setting in which we derive our friends and foes, and it is often considered to provide our defining role. It is inevitable therefore, that health can be dramatically influenced by factors within the workplace. However, we can also bring home-life conflicts and problems into the workplace. Primary care, for example, is dominated by dealing with stress-related or relationship problems, often stemming from people feeling increasingly burdened with the requirements and expectations of the workplace and of partners. This chapter explores the issues surrounding lifestyle and possible factors influencing the healthy balance of the central occupations in our life. The effects of workplace stress and the employers' attempts to reduce this are examined. Although there is the suggestion that work-based schemes to encourage a more family friendly approach for workers, it still remains the individual's choice to control how much work is allowed to interfere home life and vice versa.

The client handouts provided, encourage individuals to look at their life as a whole rather than directing 'blame' at home or at work. Take-home tasks concentrate on building self-efficacy and challenging the 'victim of the system' thinking. In addition, individuals are asked to consider the meaning of their daily occupations, and how to reintroduce that meaning while coping with an the seemingly meaningless. Getting the 'right' balance is explored with an emphasis on how too much of any one thing can be deleterious to health; conversely, too little activity which is enjoyable and relaxing can dramatically reduce the capacity to cope with the more difficult elements of life.

Importance and meaning of our daily occupations

'Every day, through their daily occupations, people create and recreate themselves and shape the world in some way'. (Wilcock, 1999, p. 77)

Many occupational scientists and occupational therapists expound the theory that the occupations which we choose, and are able to engage in are at the core of human experience and define who we are (Wilcock, 1998; Whiteford *et al.*, 2000; Christiansen and Townsend, 2004). It is, therefore, simplistic to be persuaded by even the most disaffected worker that it is solely one occupation that is instrumental in their sense of lifestyle imbalance. Indeed, it is important to include some form of competitive work or paid employment to gain a healthy occupational balance, and to promote a sense of identity and motivation (Christiansen, 1999; Whiteford, 2004). Rebeiro and Cook (1999) argue that providing opportunities for engagement in occupation is a means to improved mental health. Therefore, it is not the 'what' in what you do, but the 'why'and 'how'. Likewise, labouring in occupations that are serving no personal purpose, and that are not occupations of choice, can feel (and were used as) a form of punishment (Molineux, 2004). Indeed, some health and social care professionals, including occupational therapists, consider that health is synonymous with meaningful and purposeful activity (Molineux, 2002; Finlay, 2004).

Work as an occupation in itself can have a positive effect on health, yet when employed work becomes meaningless or senselessly repetitive and the employee feels incapacitated in performing the occupation, perceived mental health is worsened (Crist *et al.*, 2000). Employed work is also seen as a therapeutic tool for improving mental well-being in those affected by severe and enduring mental illness (Eklund *et al.*, 2004). The ability to perform to our satisfaction in our daily occupations is also influential. Withdrawal from, or changes in, our daily occupations have a significant impact on our self-perceived health and well-being (Law *et al.*, 1998).

As lifestyle imbalance has been seen to disrupt health, it can also be seen to disrupt performance; optimal occupational performance occurs with maximised 'fit' between the person, environment and occupation (Law *et al.*, 1996). In relating good health with the balance of occupations, it was found amongst a sample of the general population ($n = 146$) that reported good health significantly correlated with an equal balance of physical, mental, social and rest occupations (Wilcock *et al.*, 1997). Where the imbalance is towards sedentary occupations, there is evidence of increased risk of a number of disorders, including obesity, heart problems, diabetes and some common cancers (Hu *et al.*, 2003; Varo *et al.*, 2003).

Life beyond paid employment

Maybe, like us, you have played the game of 'What if' and applied it to winning the lottery? The answers we provide are as much a function of how we experience the different elements of work and private life, irrespective of whether we describe this latter element as 'life beyond pay', 'unpaid work', 'home' or 'life'. What is clear from the times when we have played our game is that even among people who work in the same roles in the same organisations, there are vastly different perspectives and aspirations. A sizeable group, presumably valuing what work offers to them, would return to work (or be delighted to get away from home) on Monday morning as if nothing had happened. Others laugh as they envision the range of rude displays they might use in their farewell conversation with their bosses!

The growing level of work-related stress (Wainwright and Calnan, 2002) suggests not only that there are problems with the way in which work is conducted, but also in how work and home-related factors interact. Domestic, marital and employment instability all combine to create a new scenario that is increasingly linked to worsening employee well-being. However the experience is labelled, it is clear that problems result from some perception of imbalance or discordance. This becomes 'conflict' when the demand from one domain (work or home) profoundly interferes with the other (Frone *et al.*, 1992, 1997).

Whether the expressed experience of 'conflict' represents either wisdom or whining, these issues are important. In the US, work–home conflicts were rated in the top 10 of major workplace stressors (Kelloway *et al.*, 1999). It is increasingly recognised that conflict between work and home roles can lead to mental and physical problems; it also generates poor health-related behaviours (Kivimäki *et al.*, 2002; Frone, 2003). Persistent conflict is linked to low job and life satisfaction, burnout and alcohol misuse; in its own right burnout brings emotional exhaustion, depersonalisation, reduced sense of personal accomplishment and lowered psychological well-being (Frone *et al.*, 1996; Maslach and Leiter, 1997; Perrewé *et al.*, 1999).

In contrast, positive psychology increasingly highlights the value of positive emotions (e.g. joy, optimism, confidence, excitement) for adults working in creative, problem-solving and educational activity (Paterson, 2006). In the understanding that positive emotions (e.g. excitement, creativity, optimism) are valuable not only because they displace negative emotions (e.g. anxiety, worry, disappointment), but also because they allow a shift in attention from the past to the now and the future; their role in planning and accurately predicting the future should not be understated. Collectively, there is a growing realisation that subjective medicine ('if we think it, it is real') has a biological reality – studied in psychoneuroimmunology (Kiecolt-Glaser *et al.*, 2002) and in social epidemiology (Iwachi and Berkman, 2000) – and this plays an important role in our health and well-being.

Work and non-work theories; levers for action

Recent research has proposed a broad perspective for understanding of how work and home combine. This involves using a four-quadrant approach, and overall wellness is dependent upon the type of 'spillover' based on two dimensions of effects: work–home and positive–negative (Grzywacz and Marks, 2000). Positive spill-over from work-to-home has been associated with better physical and mental health. Conversely, if that spillover is negative, it can be associated with poorer physical and mental health.

One intriguing recent theoretical development has been how some companies have intentionally created spillover effects by styling 'the firm' – and its associated actions and practices – as ones 'family' (Glynn and Wrobel, 2007). This approach is under-pinned by the idea that retaining good staff is better for business than bearing the recurrent costs associated with replacing good quality staff who leave through dissatisfaction, ill-health or active recruitment to better conditions elsewhere. Where employer concerns are linked to high levels of employee disengagement from work (affecting up to 80% of UK employees; the 20% of employees who are 'actively disengaged' cost the economy up to £37.2 billion annually: Buckingham *et al.*, 1999), the meaning of work may need to become a centre of attention.

Beyond spillover, existing theory in this area highlights three further main processes that allow work and home to play a role in adult lives. Along with 'spillover', each offers ways of thinking, and therefore ways of helping, to resolve issues where one of the two partners assumes an unwanted prominence. Individually, none of these theories fully reflect the concept and, therefore, they need to be combined to understand the work–home interface (Frone, 2003).

In 'segmentation', individuals associate each domain with specific duties and actions. Rising conflict, such as might occur when unexpected demands develop in one domain, can make it difficult to segment work and home. This can provoke feelings of lack of control, frustration and poor physical and psychological health (Perrewé *et al.*, 1999). One further theoretical perspective shows how individuals may 'compensate' commitments between the two domains. This involves reducing or expanding contributions to one domain according to those of the other (e.g. working longer hours to finance a family holiday). In family situations, unilateral decision-making based around this understanding, can fundamentally alter the nature of either work or home for others in that domain.

In border theory (Guest, 2000), emphasis is placed on everyday management of the borders between work and home. Here problems arise from the fundamental differences between values and behaviours in the distinctive domains. Border theory is helpful for understanding what and how people change to manage their border crossings. Further, where modification is possible, this is thought to reduce any potential conflict. In contrast, conflict intensifies where modification is not considered possible, because individuals are not unable, or not allowed, to become central to that domain. Border theory gives new meaning to notions of adaptability, friendliness, integration and support in both work and non-work domains.

We can add to the complexity of the factors with a role to play in determining responses to 'conflict'. Both internal and external factors determine individual approaches to reducing conflict, and even to what may constitute conflict for one person. Our individual approaches can reflect the span of perceiving, tolerating, resisting, ignoring or resolving. The options we adopt may reflect elements of personality type. Where personality is characterised by hardiness or assertiveness, we may attach different meanings to work or home (Rabin *et al.*, 1999), suggesting distinctive needs. For example, a recent Health and Safety Executive report (Daniels *et al.*, 2002) showed that individuals variously sought changes in organisational processes and managerial support or they undertook personal avoidance behaviours to manage their risk of conflict.

These response options also indicate that individuals feel more or less self-confident to adopt different approaches. Further, it is also possible that one method for resolving work–home conflict is to adopt a scatter-gun approach in the hope that a wide range of options engages affected individuals. These solutions may find their origin in the many ways in which we associate with either the work or home domains, whether *inter alia*, as mother/father, career-builder, rising star, executive, breadwinner, martyr for employee rights, workaholic or perfectionist.

Work and well-being

A strong body of literature documents that many work-related factors affect physical and psychological health. Work figures very strongly in supporting the identity of many employees; US data recently showed that American employees attribute nearly a quarter of their life satisfaction to job happiness (Grawitch *et al.*, 2007). The evidence suggests that engagement in activities and occupations that have meaning can increase motivation in people experiencing severe mental illness (Mee and Sumison, 2001). However, other studies show that features of the workplace are linked to problematic values for known cardiovascular risks, including blood pressure, cholesterol, plasma fibrinogen and catecholamines (Niedhammer *et al.*, 1998). As well as impacting on relative risk for cardiovascular morbidity and mortality (Vahtera *et al.*, 2000), stress-related factors such as repetitive work, high job demand and low social support are thought to be the greatest contributors to worsening self-reported health (Peterson, 1994; Rabin *et al.*, 1999).

Gender

Since the late 1990s, there has been a growing trend towards differentiating the needs of males and females. Under the motif of 'equal but different' a range of research evidence is showing unique gender needs. In many cases, surprisingly, this evidence directly contradicts the popular assumption of a 'health dividend' for men (White and Cash, 2004; White and Holmes, 2006). For women, issues of equity have played their role to restrict access to many forms of employment, promotional opportunities and equal pay. At a biological level, this may be evidenced by the gender-distinctive risks associated with the same blood pressure measures, waist circumferences and cholesterol values. Equally distinctive are the responses to illness, disease, emotional responses to setbacks or civil disturbances (Kiecolt-Glaser *et al.*, 2002).

Given different gender preferences for (a) communication patterns, (b) adoption of different services, (c) reasons for engagement in healthy eating, and regular exercising or (d) adopting different job roles, it is clear that life is different in many important ways for the majority of men as compared to women. While the most consistent evidence of what causes conflict is found in women (Benavides *et al.*, 2002), a growing body of evidence also shows that these issues are becoming prominent in men (Emslie *et al.*, 2004). For these reasons, work–home conflict can be seen as being linked to different sex roles. For example, for women, key factors might include combining having children and being in a senior position. In men, working longer and typically unsociable hours may be more important factors. Irrespective of gender, working long work hours can increase the risk of developing hypertension, which then will require lifestyle modification of the established risk factors such as smoking, diabetes, obesity and sedentary lifestyle (Yang *et al.*, 2006). Single-person parenting or caring can add extra work requiring completion of a 'second shift' upon returning home from paid work (Hochschild and Machung, 1989).

Stereotypically, women are the main support for family and children, and balancing these 'home' and 'work' responsibilities can impair individual health (Burke and Greenglass, 1999; Kar *et al.*, 1999). Conflict worsens when important activities occur at the same time but they are in different venues; this can lead to increased absenteeism that affects colleagues and employers alike. When conflict persists to produce burnout, two possibilities ensue: the first is prolonged absenteeism, the second is presenteeism, which involves working while unfit (Koopman *et al.*, 2004). At work, burnout-presenteeism reduces work performance and lowers job satisfaction (Rabin *et al.*, 1999). Recent estimates suggest that lost work performance attributable to absenteeism represented 2% of losses, compared to 63% for presenteeism (Hemp, 2004).

Other studies suggest that womens' responsiveness to unexpected work demands is difficult in the face of numerous home factors, including (1) having more (especially young) children, (2) having partners with high work commitments or (3) having a low total home income (e.g. Shelton, 1990; Peterson, 1994; Burke and Greenglass, 1999; Kar *et al.*, 1999; Rabin *et al.*, 1999). These may be useful indicators of possible 'targets' for marketing of support services. Staff with such home demands may experience particular difficulties with work-related travel and international teleconferencing.

Importantly, conflict may emerge as a result of a strong sense of 'caring', although it is important to appreciate that position within a company influences how much autonomy can be employed, and this is important in determining the presence of conflict. For women, the stereotypical view is that work interferes more, and with greater impact, on home issues than vice versa. This may result from the home domain having the most permeable boundaries (Frone *et al.*, 1992). For many employees, career progression may hinge on fitting in with longer hours work cultures. This appreciation may underpin the frustrations that some employees may have when their other commitments do not allow such flexibility.

General themes for interventions

As with most health-related issues, it is possible to establish primary, secondary and tertiary prevention approaches. In keeping with most interventions, we imagine that change will mostly be enacted after a problem has emerged; certainly, the link to work–life conflict suggests a *post hoc* approach. Existing literature shows only limited successes from workplace interventions (Schaufeli and Buunk, 2003), while Fletcher (2003) makes a convincing case for attention (and change) to begin with the individual. We make no claims for the efficacy of any intervention, such as exercising, to be better than any other (e.g. relaxation, meditation or diet change) for restoring life balance. Further, the lack of empirical evidence may reflect the ongoing problem with translating laboratory-based interventions into the free-form world of daily life. What does seem clear is that satisfaction with work remains connected to key factors: influence in the job world, self-determination over workplace and practice, a sense of the meaningfulness of one's work and workplace cooperation and fellowship (Gardell, 1981).

Since most people only become concerned about lost balance once it is lost, it may be useful to consider the wide range of options that facilitate improved coping. Skinner and Zimmer-Gembeck (2007) recently reviewed the coping literature, summarising the options as 'instrumental action, problem-solving, support-seeking, distraction, escape, opposition and social withdrawal' (p. 121).

Workplace interventions

Workplace programmes and policies can facilitate work–life balance by acknowledging the competing demands of many employees' complex lives. Since growing conflict between work and other responsibilities can diminish the quality of both work and home life for employees, this can also lead to reduced productivity, absenteeism and increased turnover. In contrast, efforts to help employees improve their work–life balance can improve morale, increase job satisfaction and strengthen commitment to the company/organisation. In addition, the organisation may reap benefits in terms of increased productivity and reducted absenteeism, presenteeism and employee turnover. One recent US study highlighted how every dollar spent on providing a multidimensional workplace health promotion programme was rewarded with over $15 of cost savings (Aldana *et al.*, 2005). Summaries show absenteeism savings to the value of £2.50 for every pound spent on the interventions (Kreis and Bödeker, 2004).

A wide variety of approaches can be used, individually or in combination, to alter the subjective elements that may lead to better work–life balance. Recent work in counselling for health behaviour change has highlighted the extra value of simultaneous counselling for behavioural changes over sequential change (Hyman *et al.*, 2007). However, there are also principles for supporting preventive programmes (Nation *et al.*, 2003) and these may be readily applied to work–life balance. Applications are sufficiently general to allow for modification to local circumstances: (1) comprehensive content, (2) varied teaching approaches, (3) sufficient doses (including follow-ups), (4) theory driven (to generate empirical outcomes), (5) positive relationships, (6) appropriately timed (to maximise impact), (7) socioculturally relevant (to capitalise on group strengths and needs), (8) outcome evaluation and (9) well-trained staff. These are provided in a template (see Handout 3.1) which you can use to plan new, or refine existing, interventions.

The perception of the workplace is as important as the reality in determining the psychological health of the employee. Autonomy underpins definitions of what qualifies as a work–life balance strategy, as employees seek to coordinate and integrate these elements of their lives (Felstead *et al.*, 2002). Further, the psychologically healthy workplace often demonstrates other practices, including both top-down and bottom-up communication patterns that facilitate employee involvement, employee growth and development (opportunities for learning and self-improvement); health and safety and employee recognition (attention and rewards) (Grawitch *et al.*, 2007). Programmes and policies that can promote work–life balance include: flexible work arrangements, such as flexitime and telecommuting (allowing more work from home); assistance with childcare; eldercare benefits; support for personal financial issues; benefits for domestic partners and flexible leave options. A key issue is to encourage all qualified employees to adopt and use such services.

In workplaces, time management is often seen as a viable solution. While this may be effective where people are time inefficient, for others this is simply irrelevant given their outstanding pre-existing skills in managing multiple competing demands (Bryson *et al.*, 2007). For them, expressions relating to 'lack of time' may be more related to their commitment to multiple roles and tasks, rather than to time itself. In this understanding, existing support for time management may be better refocused on how carers determine and change their home and work priorities. Indeed, for many, home is a location for completing numerous tasks, often unrewarded or where they are taken-for-granted. Where individuals hold strong, but unrealised, aspirational values for home life, work may become an important substitute venue for recognition, affiliation, achievement and reward. Indeed, damage to supportive relationships built between colleagues is often an unacknowledged casualty of the re-organisation and downsizing practices that have become commonplace since the 1990s. Having a friend at work is one key indicator of high-level engagement (Buckingham and Coffman, 1999). At another level, work may provide an important venue for connecting to others; low social connectedness worsens health outcomes across a range of scenarios (Berkman and Glass, 2000; McNeill *et al.*, 2006).

Work-based relationships are clearly important both in initiating and resolving some conflicts. For example, occasional lapses in empathy from colleagues at all levels in an organisation can lead them to behave in ways that add to conflict. Among part-time staff, their 'visibility' may become reduced, paradoxically creating exposure to work practices they had sought to avoid by working fewer hours. Solutions to such problems may lie in developing assertiveness skills in communicating with work colleagues.

Given the diverse set of influences on work satisfaction, it is clear that home is likely be similarly complex, suggesting that eclectic intervention approaches may be wise. Ford (1992) highlights that to be effective in any element of life requires four components: biological capacity, responsive environment, self-motivation and skills to (1) construct and then (2) carry out a plan. The mosaic of needs demonstrated, or even perceived, by an individual is likely to be highly dynamic and in need of follow-up. To build interventions based on these factors, it is wise to begin by understanding that there is likely to be a considerable level of interaction between these factors. Here we focus on two factors: skills and self-motivation.

Skills to (1) construct and then (2) carry out a plan

Fletcher (2003) emphasises that it may be easier – and wiser – to focus change attempts on individuals for at least two reasons: first, it may be easier to change an individual than a whole culture (e.g. workplaces, family value systems) and, second, any changes in a culture will always be mediated by the outlook of the individual who interprets those changes. One simple example is the willingness of individuals to create, take or negotiate me-time during the work day and in the home. In Ford's conceptualisation, 'skill' has two important components, the second of which highlights that although individuals can build plans, the plan is only as effective as its capacity to be sustained through tough times. Plans based on existing personal strengths capitalise on pre-existing self-confidence and self-confidence is one of the strongest predictors of sustained self-change. Adopting 'implementation intentions' (Gollwitzer and Brandstätter, 1997), where individuals write their plan and specify a date for taking their first steps, helps people who have already expressed a wish to change.

Relapse prevention theory (Marlatt and Gordon, 1985) emphasises the value of planning for set-back moments, particularly for continuing to thrive beyond what might be considered as the 'blow out moment' within any change plan. Psychological resilience (paradoxically described as 'Knowing what to do when you do not know what to do') may be another element to develop within careful planning. The self-assessment tool (Handout 3.2) highlights a number of attitudinal and behavioural factors that may be addressed to build resilience.

At an individual level there are a number of skills that can be deployed to reduce exposure to stress-creating events and settings, to modify (or minimise) negative responses to events or to avoid exposure altogether. Counselling literature can be used to identify different approaches that help individuals to develop – and verbalise – changes that suit their lifestyles, skills and needs. These include motivational interviewing (Britt *et al.*, 2003; Knight *et al.*, 2006), solution focused techniques (Mackey-Jones and McKenna, 2002) and cognitive behavioural therapy approaches. While there are advantages to delivery based on trained professionals, self-help evidence suggests that the techniques associated with these approaches can be employed to good effect (Scogin *et al.*, 1990) even by non-professional counsellors (e.g. McKenna and Mackey-Jones, 2004). Many of these approaches simply generate a range of options for change, support ongoing change or provide opportunities for developing and refining specific skills.

For example, cognitive-behaviour-based techniques focus on identifying thoughts that might create problems. Building a plan for alternative interpretations of events may be an important first step in changing these responses. Rehearsing pre-planned positive thoughts (e.g. 'I belong in this job') can be connected to the occurence of every-day events to a common action, such as hearing the phone ring.

Nelson-Jones (1997) offers a wide range of skills that can be adapted to suit most workplaces, many of which focus on how to think creatively and positively in a range of different circumstances. Sport psychology, so often focused on high-level performance in stressful environments, emphasises the psychological skills that may help adapt to environments that are overly demanding and include psychological blunting ('It doesn't matter to me'), emotional coping ('I've felt worse, I can cope') or problem-based coping ('I've been here before and I know how to handle it'). Goal-setting (setting behavioural targets for the future), imagery (positive day dreaming) and positive reinforcement (providing rewards) are other techniques that collectively shift cognitions and that support new directions for behaviour that may benefit life either at work or home.

Consistent with Thompson and Bunderson (2001), Guest (2002), Mackey-Jones and McKenna (2002) and Covey (2004) discuss that a shift in mindset may be an important way to establish better life balance. Both Guest (2002) and Covey (2004) highlight the value in shifting the unit of analysis from time to value. In effect, they each recommend – in varying ways – the importance of dedicating time to things that give life meaning. For the women in Mackey-Jones and McKenna (2004), solution-focused approaches helped them identify the need for, and ways to use, 'me-time'. Clearly, the challenge that results from such calls is that finding meaning is exactly the problem; Caproni (2004) underlines the elusiveness of mind-changing in her title, 'Work/Life Balance: You Can't Get There from Here'.

Self-motivation

Self-motivation as described here emphasises that individuals motivate themselves according to their needs, aspirations, commitments and life plans. Importantly, health practitioners may have missed an important 'trick' here. Psychology increasingly underlines that individuals motivate themselves, making this an important feature in delivering more relevant interventions. While health may be a motive for many people (although effectiveness in generating change is often best developed among people whose health functioning is already compromised), further – and often substantially more important – motives should be considered. Techniques borrowed from solution-focused interventions may be readily adopted for this purpose. Self-motivation also has a powerful role to play in determining the appeal of existing programme provision. Using the case of a 'typical' working man, we invite you to compare the respective appeal of yoga over weight-training or five-a-side soccer. At a wider level, self-motivation influences whether home or work is considered as the ideal venue for change and, within that, what approaches might be undertaken.

This underlines the need to adopt methods where individuals can establish their personal motives. For example, career progression may be a strong motive for one person, whereas for another being a 'good dad' or 'good mum' may create incentive for change. At another level, for individuals from traditionally hard-to-reach communities, simply listening to their life narratives may represent an important time for them to connect with motives that they had not yet seen for themselves (Frank, 1995). There can be few more powerful events than that which reveals a whole new direction in life (see Advice box 3.2).

Conclusion

This chapter has detailed the processes by which work–non-work conflict may arise. On the basis of a range of theoretical perspectives, the mechanisms that both lead to, and show the pathway from, this conflict have been addressed. Although there are numerous approaches that can reduce conflict, this experience can be seen as being individualised, which justifies individualised support. However, where systems and where custom-and-practice are seen as problematic, corporate policy needs to be developed to address and support positive interpersonal behaviour. This can be justified on a number of grounds from improving individual health, reducing staff turnover and increasing work performance.

References

Aldana, S. G., Merrill, R. M., Price, K., Hardy, A. and Hager, R. (2005). Financial impact of a comprehensive workplace health promotion program. *Preventive Medicine*, 40: 131–137.

Benavides, F. G., Benach, J. and Muntaner, C. (2002). Psychosocial risk factors at the workplace: is there enough evidence to establish reference values? *Journal of Epidemiology and Community Health*, 56: 244–245.

Berkman, L. F. and Glass, T. (2000). Social integration, social networks, social support and health. In Berkman, L. F. and Kawachi, I. (eds) *Social Epidemiology*. New York, Oxford University Press, Chapter 7, pp. 137–173.

Britt, E., Hudson, S. M. and Blampied, N. M. (2003). Motivational interviewing in health settings: a review. *Patient Education and Counseling*, 53: 147–155.

Bryson, L., Warner-Smith, P., Brown, P. and Fray, L. (2007). Managing the work–life roller-coaster; private stress or public health issue? *Social Science and Medicine*, 65: 1142–1153.

Buckingham, M. and Coffman, C. (1999). *First Break All the Rules: What the World's Greatest Managers Do Differently*. London, Simon & Schuster.

Burke, R. J. and Greenglass, E. R. (1999). Hospital restructuring, work–family conflict and psychological burnout among nursing staff. *Journal of Occupational Health Psychology*, 4: 327–336.

Caproni, P. J. (2004). Work/life balance: you can't get there from here. *Journal of Applied Behavioural Science*, 40: 208–218.

Christiansen, C. H. (1999). Defining lives: occupation as identity: an essay on competence, coherence, and the creation of meaning. *The American Journal of Occupational Therapy*, 53: 547–558.

Christiansen, C. H. and Townsend, E. A. (2004). An introduction to occupation. In Christiansen, C. H. and Townsend, E. A. (eds) *Introduction to Occupation: The Art and Science of Living*. Upper Saddle River, NJ, Prentice-Hall, pp. 1–28.

Covey, S. (2004). *The 8th Habit: From Effectiveness to Greatness*. London, Simon & Schuster.

Crist, P. H., Davis, C. G. and Coffin, P. S. (2000). The effects of employment and mental health status on the balance of work, play/leisure, self-care, and rest. *Occupational Therapy in Mental Health*, 15: 27–42.

Daniels, K., Harris, C. and Briner, R. B. (2002). *Understanding the Risks of Stress: A Cognitive Approach.* Health and Safety Executive, HMSO, Norwich.

Eklund, M., Hansson, L. and Ahlqvist, C. (2004). The importance of work as compared to other forms of daily occupations for wellbeing and functioning among persons with long-term mental illness. *Community Mental Health Journal*, 40 (5): 465–477.

Emslie, C., Hunt, K. and Macintyre, S. (2004). Gender, work-home conflict, and minor morbidity amongst white-collar bank employees in the UK. *International Journal of Behavioural Medicine*, 11: 127–134.

Felstead, A., Jewson, N., Phizacklea, A. and Walters, S. (2002). Opportunities to work at home in the context of work–life balance. *Human Resources Management Journal*, 12: 54–77.

Finlay, L. (2004). *The Practice of Psychosocial Occupational Therapy*, 3rd edition. Cheltenham, Nelson Thornes.

Fletcher, B. C. (2003). The FIT approach to work stress and health. In Schabracq, M. J., Winnubst, J. A. M. and Cooper, C. L. (eds) *The Handbook of Work and Health Psychology*, 2nd edition. Chichester, John Wiley, Chapter 26, pp. 546–568.

Frank, A. W. (1995). *The Wounded Storyteller*. Chicago, IL, University of Chicago Press.

Frone, M. R. (2003). Work–family balance. In Quick, J. C. and Tetrick, L. E. (eds) *Handbook of Occupational Health Psychology*. Washington, DC, American Psychological Association.

Frone, M. R., Russell, M. and Barnes, G. M. (1996). Work–family conflict, gender, and health-related outcomes: a study of employed parents in two community samples. *Journal of Occupational Psychology*, 1: 57–69.

Frone, M. R., Russell, M. and Cooper, M. L. (1992). Prevalence of work–family conflict: are work and family boundaries asymmetrically permeable? *Journal of Organisational Behaviour*, 13: 723–729.

Frone, M. R., Yardley, J. K. and Markel, K. S. (1997). Developing and testing an integrative model of the work–family interface. *Journal of Vocational Behaviour*, 50: 145–167.

Glynn, M. A. and Wrobel, K. (2007). My family, my firm: how familial relationships function as endogenous organisational resources. In Dutton, J. E. and Ragins, B. R. (eds) *Exploring Positive Relationships at Work: Building a Theoretical and Research Foundation*. NJ, Lawrence Erlbaum, Chapter 17, pp. 307–323.

Gollwitzer, P. M. and Brandstätter, V. (1997). Implementation intentions and effective goal pursuit. *Journal of Personality and Social Psychology*, 73: 186–199.

Grawitch, M., Gottschalk, M. and Munz, D. C. (2007). The path to a healthy workplace: a critical review linking healthy workplace practices, employee well-being, and organizational improvements. *Consulting Psychology Journal: Practice and Research*, 58: 129–147.

Grzywacz, J. G. and Marks, N. F. (2000). Reconceptualising the work–family interface: an ecological perspective on the correlates of positive and negative spillover between work and family. *Journal of Occupational Health Psychology*, 5: 111–126.

Guest, D. E. (2002). Perspectives on the study of work–life balance. *Social Sciences Information*, 41: 255–279.

Guest, D. E. and Conway, N. (2000). *The Psychological Contract in the Public Sector*. London, Chartered Institute of Personnel and Development (CIPD).

Hemp, P. (2004). Presenteeism: at work – but out of it. *Harvard Business Review*, 82: 49–58.

Hu, F. B., Li, T.Y., Colditz, G. A., Walter, C., Willett, P. H. and Manson, J. A. E. (2003). Television watching and other sedentary behaviours in relation to risk of obesity and Type 2 diabetes mellitus in women. *JAMA*, 289: 1785–1791.

Hyman, D. J., Pavlik, V. N., Taylor, W. C., Goodrick, G. K. and Moye, L. (2007). Simultaneous vs sequential counseling for multiple behaviour change. *Archives of Internal Medicine*, 167: 1152–1158.

Kar, S. B., Pascual, C. A. and Chickering, K. L. (1999). Empowerment of women for health promotion: a meta-analysis. *Social Science and Medicine*, 49: 1431–1460.

Kelloway, E. K., Gottleib, B. H. and Barham, L. (1999). The source, nature and direction of work and family conflict; a longitudinal investigation. *Journal of Occupational Health Psychology*, 4: 337–346.

Kiecolt-Glaser, J. K., McGuire, L., Robles, T. F. and Glaser, R. (2002). Emotions, morbidity and mortality: new perspectives from psychoneuroimmunology. *Annual Review of Psychology*, 53: 83–107.

Kivimäki, M., Leino-Arjas, P., Luukkonen, R., Riihimäki, H., Vahtera, J. and Kirjonen, J. (2002). Work stress and risk of cardiovascular mortality: prospective cohort study of industrial employees. *British Medical Journal*, 325: 857–861.

Knight, K. M., McGowan, L., Dickens, C. and Bundy, C. (2006). A systematic review of motivational interviewing in physical health care settings. *British Journal of Health Psychology*, 11: 319–332.

Koopman, C., Pelletier, K. R., Murray, J. F. *et al.* (2004). Stanford presenteeism scale: health status and employee productivity. *Journal of Occupational and Environmental Medicine*, 44: 14–20.

Kreis, J. and Böedeker, W. (2004). *Health-related and Economic Benefits of Workplace Health Promotion and Prevention: Summary of the Scientific Evidence*. Essen, BKK Bundesverband.

Law, M., Steinwender, S. and Leclair, L. (1998). Occupation, health and well being. *Canadian Journal of Occupational Therapy*, 65(2): 81–91.

Mackey-Jones, W. and McKenna, J. (2002). Women and work–home conflict: a dual paradigm approach. *Health Education*, 102: 249–259.

Marlatt, G. A. and Gordon, J. R. (1985). *Relapse Prevention*. New York, Guilford.

Maslach, C. and Leiter, M. P. (1997). *The Truth about Burnout*. San Francisco, CA, Jossey-Bass.

McKenna, J. and Mackey-Jones, W. (2004). How solution-focused therapy helps women through work-home conflict. *Health Education*, 104: 132–142.

McNeill, L. H., Kreuter, M. W. and Subramanian, S. V. (2006). Social environment and physical activity: a review of concepts and evidence. *Social Science and Medicine*, 63: 1011–1022.

Molineux, M. (2002). The age of occupation: an opportunity to be seized. *Mental Health Occupational Therapy*, 7: 12–14.

Molineux, M. (2004). Occupation in occupational therapy: a labour in vain? In Molineux, M. (ed.) *Occupation for Occupational Therapists*. Oxford, Blackwell Publishing, pp. 1–14.

Nation, M., Crusto, C., Wabdersman, A. *et al.* (2003). What works in prevention: principles of effective prevention programs. *American Psychologist*, 58: 449–456.

Nelson-Jones, R. (1997). *Using Your Mind: Creative Thinking for Work and Business Success*. London, Cassell.

Niedhammer, I., Goldberg, M., Leclerc, A., David, S., Bugel, I. and Landre, M.-F. (1998). Psychosocial work environment and cardiovascular risk factors in an occupational cohort in France. *Journal of Epidemiology and Community Health*, 52: 93–100.

Paterson, C. (2006). *A Primer in Positive Psychology*. Oxford, Oxford University Press.

Perrewé, P. L., Hochwarter, W. A. and Kiewitz, C. (1999). Value attainment: an explanation for the negative effects of work–family conflict on job and life satisfaction. *Journal of Occupational Health Psychology*, 4: 318–326.

Peterson, C. L. (1994). Work factors and stress: a critical review. *International Journal of Health Sciences*, 24: 495–519.

Rabin, S., Feldman, D. and Kaplan, Z. (1999). Stress and intervention strategies in mental health professionals. *British Journal of Medical Psychology*, 72: 159–169.

Rebeiro, K. L. and Cook, J. V. (1999). Opportunity, not prescription: an exploratory study of the experience of occupational engagement. *Canadian Journal of Occupational Therapy*, 66: 176–187.

Schaufel, W. B. and Buunk, B. P. (2003). Burnout: an overview of 25 years of research and theorising. In Schabracq, M. J., Winnubst, J. A. M. and Cooper, C. L. (eds) *The Handbook of Work and Health Psychology*, 2nd edition. Chichester, John Wiley, Chapter 19, pp. 383–425.

Scogin, F., Bynum, J., Stephens, G. and Calhoon, S. (1990). Efficacy of self-administered treatment programs: meta-analytic review. *Professional Psychology: Research and Practice*, 21: 42–47.

Shelton, B. (1990). The distribution of household tasks; does a wife's employment status make a difference? *Journal of Family Issues*, 11: 115–135.

Skinner, E. A. and Zimmer-Gembeck, M. J. (2007). The development of coping. *Annual Review of Psychology*, 58: 119–144.

Thompson, J. A. and Bunderson, J. S. (2001). Work–nonwork conflict and the phenomenology of time: beyond the balance metaphor. *Work and Occupations*, 28: 17–39.

Vahtera, J., Kivimäki, M., Pentti, J. and Theorell, T. (2000). Effect of change in the psychosocial work environment on sickness absence: a seven year follow up of initially healthy employees. *Journal of Epidemiology Community Health*, 54: 484–493.

Varo, J. J., Martínez-González, M. A., de Irala-Estévez, J., Kearney, J., Gibney, M. and Martínez, J. A. (2003). Distribution and determinants of sedentary lifestyles in the European Union. *International Journal of Epidemiology*, 32: 138–146.

Wainwright, D. and Calnan, M. (2002). *Work and Stress: The Making of a Modern Epidemic*. Buckingham, Open University.

White, A. K. and Cash, K. (2004). The state of men's health in Western Europe. *Journal of Men's Health and Gender*, 1: 60–66.

White, A. K. and Holmes, M. (2006). Patterns of morbidity across 44 countries among men and women aged 15–44. *Journal of Men's Health and Gender*, 3: 139–151.

Whiteford, G. (2004). When people cannot participate: occupational deprivation. In Christiansen, C. H. and Townsend, E. A. (eds) *Introduction to Occupation: The Art and Science of Living*. Upper Saddle River, NJ, Prentice-Hall, pp. 221–242.

Whiteford, G., Townsend, E. and Hocking, C. (2000). Reflections on a renaissance of occupation. *Canadian Journal of Occupational Therapy*, 67: 61–69.

Wilcock, A. (1998). Reflections on doing, being, and becoming. *Canadian Journal of Occupational Therapy*, 65: 248–256.

Wilcock, A. (1999). Creating self and shaping the world. *Australian Occupational Therapy Journal*, 46: 77–88.

Wilcock, A., Chelin, M., Hall, M. *et al.* (1997). The relationship between occupational balance and health: a pilot study. *Occupational Therapy International*, 1: 17–30.

Yang, H., Schnall, P. L., Jauregui, M., Su, T. -S. and Baker, D. (2006). Work hours and self-reported hypertension among working people in California. *Hypertension*, 48: 1–2.

Key websites

http://humanresources.about.com
www.mindtools.com
www.motivation-tools.com/workplace
www.resiliencycenter.com

Note on Advice boxes

Advice boxes 3.1–3.4 offer specific advice based on the evidence that has been presented, they complement and accompany the handouts that are provided, which can be photocopied.

The lifestyle circle should be individually created, and it merely requires a blank sheet of paper with a large circle, which the client is advised to divide-up in accordance to the instructions (Handout 3.4).

All of the following handouts and advice boxes can be found as individual pdfs on the website at www.blackwellpublishing.com/thew

Advice box 3.1 Helping people create a more satisfying work–life balance

In helping people create a more satisfying work–life balance, it can be tempting to blame the workplace, and therefore, retire or go on extended sick leave, thereby avoiding the workplace and creating more time to devote to home life. Handout 3.1 will help identify the potential of any workplace for helping individuals to resolve unwanted conflict between work and non-work life. This we have seen is not necessarily as quickly resolved as may be assumed. Clients may need to consider the benefits of work. Handouts 3.2 and 3.3 can help in questioning the usefulness of turning away from meaningful occupation merely to end up filling the hours with meaningless daily chores.

With work taking up many hours of our waking lives, it may be useful for the therapist to ask the client to identify the enjoyable elements of work, for example friendships, routine, achievement, recognition for work achieved, and so on, which make the working day more positive. Encouragement of frequent breaks from repetitive and often boring tasks can make the working day more relaxing and enjoyable. This could be achieved by using Handouts 3.2, 3.3 and 3.4 to identify personal coping strategies and time spent in the varying occupations of the day.

Advice box 3.2 Listening to the life narrative

Listening to the life narrative may help the individual to recognise the elements of their life that give most meaning; this is best done by asking questions such as 'what are you like at your best?'. This is a more positive framework than exploring the dissatisfying elements, and reflecting on the positive promotes facilitation of positive change.

This may then help facilitate the realisation that spending hours agonising over work issues whilst at home, when the most satisfying and defining life role is being a mother, is wasting precious time engaging and enjoying the more meaningful occupations, such as spending time playing with the children.

Advice box 3.3 Analysing daily routines

Challenging the status quo: the daily routine can be analysed (using Handout 3.3) to identify the occupations that are least or most enjoyable/satisfying. However, changing the current routine can be difficult. By challenging the thoughts that can act as barriers to change (Handout 3.4), the client can start to make small changes that can grow to more substantive change (Handout 3.5). By encouraging gradual adaptation of the daily routine to incorporate more hours spent in meaningful and enjoyable occupations, the goal of a healthier life balance can be achieved.

Advice box 3.4 Returning to work

It may be helpful to use the evidence provided in this chapter to help individuals to return to the workplace after a prolonged absence, by informing the employer the benefits of introducing more sociable and family focused terms of employment. The reward for the workplace is a more productive work force. This can be in the form of return to work recommendations or report. The employee can also be involved in the 'new' return to work guidelines, and can start to introduce a more balanced and healthy work routine, incorporating breaks, exercise and relaxing behaviours. Encouraging flexible hours can help take the pressure off domestic routines such as getting children to school or working from home. In addition, assertiveness strategies and in-house training schemes should be encouraged to help the individual face the dilemmas of the workplace, rather than avoid them with sick leave.

Handout 3.1 Preventing work–life conflict

Revising your provision or planned intervention

	Score for current provision or plan (10 is excellent)	**Comments**
How comprehensive is the content?	/10	
What are our teaching approaches?	/10	
Are there sufficient doses (including follow-ups)?	/10	
What theory is driving this?	/10	
How do we develop positive relationships?	/10	
What is it timed with (to maximise impact)?	/10	
How is it socio-culturally relevant?	/10	
How will I assess effectiveness?	/10	
How well have we trained our staff?	/10	

Source: From Nation *et al*. (2003).

Look over your scores. Where scores are less than 9 reconsider your plan or your current provision. It is NOT likely to be effective. Refine your plan until you achieve a (genuine) score of 9+ for every item.

Handout 3.2 How resilient are you?

How do you react to life's difficulties? Healthy, resilient people have stress-resistant personalities and learn valuable lessons from rough experiences. They often rebound even stronger from major setbacks.

Take the quiz. Use the boxes to rate yourself (1 = not at all like me, 5 = very like me) on the following:

Add up your scores; higher numbers show greater resilience.

In a crisis or chaotic situation, I calm myself and focus on taking useful actions.	
I am usually optimistic. I see difficulties as temporary and expect to overcome.	
I can tolerate high levels of ambiguity and uncertainty about situations.	
I adapt quickly to new developments. I am good at bouncing back from difficulties.	
I am playful. I find the humour in tough situations, and can laugh at myself.	
I recover emotionally from losses and setbacks. I have friends to talk with. I can express my feelings to others and ask for help. Feelings of anger, loss and discouragement do not last long.	
I feel self-confident, appreciate myself and have a healthy concept of myself.	
I am curious and ask questions. I want to know how things work and to try new ways of doing things.	
I learn valuable lessons from my own experiences and those of others.	
I am good at solving problems. I can be creative or use my common sense.	
I make things work well. I am often asked to lead groups and projects.	

I am very flexible. I feel comfortable with my complexity. I am optimistic and pessimistic, trusting and cautious, unselfish and selfish, and so forth.	
I am always myself, but I change depending on the situation.	
I prefer to work without a written job description. I do well when I am free to do what I think is best in each situation.	
I 'read' people well and trust my intuition.	
I am a good listener. I have good empathy skills.	
I do not judge others and adapt to different personality styles.	
I am very durable. I hold up well during tough times. I have an independent spirit underneath my cooperative way of working with others.	
I have become stronger and better through difficult experiences.	
I convert bad into good luck and find advantages in bad experiences.	

Add up your scores; higher numbers show greater resilience.

Handout 3.3 Lifestyle – getting the right balance for health

This handout is designed to challenge your perception of your own life balance, and to help identify how to make changes that can improve your work–life balance to increase well-being and prevent health-induced breakdowns.

Is it as simple as going part time at work, or even retiring? If life was as simple as cutting the amount of time we spent at work, and then finding our life dramatically improves, then most of us would not work!

There are studies which indicate that retirement does not necessarily lead to fulfilment and pleasure-filled pastimes. Indeed, some suggest that retirement can be stressful; this could be attributed to the fact that paid employment can mean much more than a means for living.

In examining our daily life occupations, we can find that boredom can lead to psychological problems; in contrast, meaningful activity or occupation can actually define who we are. People often refer to themselves by their job titles or roles in life, such as 'I'm a nurse', 'I'm a teacher' or 'I'm a full time mum/stay at home dad'.

Time to get 'real'. By charting exactly how much of your day you spend on which activity, you can start to realistically see where in your life you can make a change. There are no fantastic solutions, but if you were to try and adopt the following strategies, your life should be more evenly balanced between the activities that are healthy for you and those that can be making you tired, stressed or low, and you could look towards improving your heath for the present and the future.

Creating a balanced lifestyle. No one should feel that they 'ought' to have a more balanced lifestyle, it should be your own choice, and this is YOUR life, not someone else's. However, there are certain requirements and expectations in being an employee, a parent, a partner, a daughter/son that make demands on your time and, therefore, on your life. These need to be balanced with other elements that make you feel positive and relaxed.

Handout 3.4 The lifestyle circle

Consider a pie chart: (Draw a circle on a piece of paper, see example below)

Step 1. Number all the activities and occupations that you engage in, for example 1 = housework, 2 = reading with the children, 3 = going out on family trip, 4 = travelling to work, or write next to each segment.

Step 2. Each day, roughly divide up your circle into 'pie' segments in approximate sized chunks per activity and put the number in the segment.

Step 3. Consider how you felt overall during the activity, did you feel relaxed, stressed, tired , or did you feel pleasure? Mark-up the segment using the following as a guide: horizontal lines = pleasure, black = stressed, hatched lines = calm/relaxed, grey = angry/frustrated, circles = sense of achievement, dots = bored, blank = no emotion.

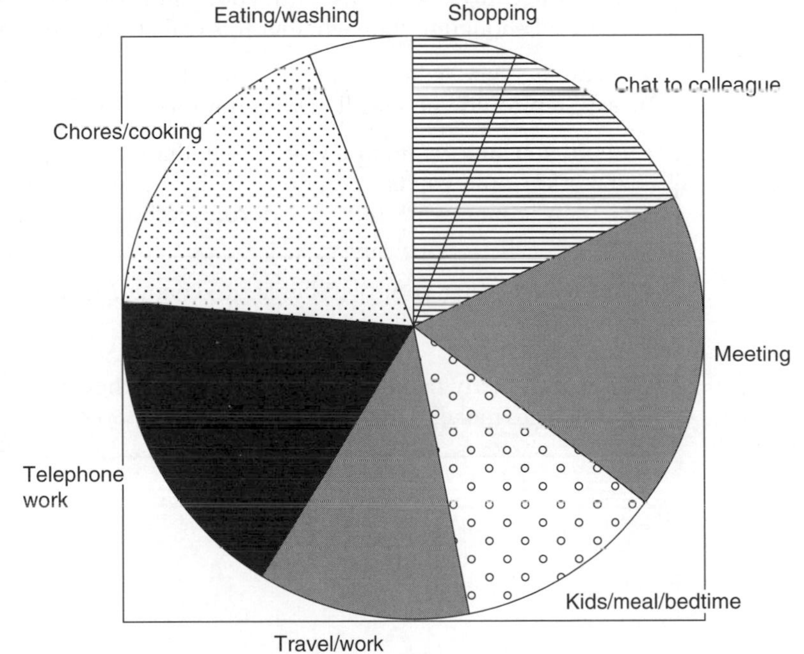

Handout 3.4 Continued

Analysing your lifestyle circles

Complete each pie chart in this manner in Handout 3.4, for a week, then sit back and consider how your life looks.

- Is it all greys and blacks? Do you see that some activities make you feel more stressed than others?
- Do you have many repetitive activities, for example, watching TV, of which only a few hours a week actually give you pleasure? How balanced are the numbers? Do you have, for example, an excess of household chores? Do you lack a social life?
- Consider each of the activities and change those that are stressful, boring or you have an excess of. It may be most appropriate to do this with your partner, a good friend, and so on, as they could challenge you on what to change and how to change it.
- If there was one thing that you would like to do differently, what would it be? Now list all the possible ways that you could make this change a reality, and discuss with your family or friend, as they know you well enough to state whether it is realistic to achieve.
- If you are very sedentary in your life, then, for example, what one, easy step could you take that would improve this?
- Could you take the stairs at work rather than the lift? Could you walk to work? Could you take your bike to the local shop? Housework can be seen to be a work out. Could you see this as an opportunity to exercise rather than a chore?
- Are you creating your own barrier to change? Is it easier to stay as you are?

However, many people get to a crisis before they consider that they would like to make changes to their life.

Handout 3.5 Achieving a more balanced lifestyle

- List what you would like to do more of.
- List what you would like to do less of.

Example

What I would like to do more of	What I would like to do less of
Meeting with my friends in the evenings	Housework
Going out for evening meals	Eating convenience foods
Going for a swim	Watching TV

What are the barriers preventing you from doing more of what you want and less of what you do not want. Discuss ways to lift the barriers with your partner/friend/therapist

Barriers

Cannot afford to eat/ social nights out	cannot afford a cleaner
Tired after work	too tired to cook decent meals
No one to go swimming with	nothing other than TV to do

Lifting barriers. Now by examining the barriers, what *can you*, not your boss, partner or friend, do towards making one small change to lift the barriers? Start with very simple changes.

Example. 'I could ask neighbour if they fancy coming for a swim to local pool straight after work, it doesn't cost much. Jacket potatoes are cheap, and healthy, could put those in for tea while I play with the children.'

Sometimes, just taking stock of how your life 'looks' with the pie charts can start to allow you to feel you have more control over the things you can change, to help you cope with the things you cannot, small changes towards a more enjoyable life will have a positive impact on your health.

Section B

LIVING WITH LIFESTYLE PROBLEMS

4. *Impact of Lifestyle on Back Pain*

Jamie Bell

Introduction

Most people will experience an episode of low back pain (LBP) during their life (Papageorgiou *et al.*, 1995), and for many this becomes a recurrent event (Croft *et al.*, 1998). Whilst some individuals will continue to function with pain, the lifestyle of many is adversely affected; disability, work-loss and care-seeking are just a few outcomes linked to LBP. Thus, the socio-economic impact of this problem on industrialised countries is substantial (van Tulder *et al.*, 2000). Despite advances in technology, the pathology and anatomical source responsible for LBP cannot be identified in the vast majority of cases, and those afflicted tend to reach a pain-free state, irrespective of whether or not they receive treatment (Pengel *et al.*, 2003). This has resulted in a move away from searching for a treatable cause for LBP, towards a more integrated biopsychosocial approach. This approach is supported by evidence that physical and often lifestyle-related factors can explain the onset of symptoms, with psychosocial factors dictating the subsequent course of LBP. Therefore, by understanding these factors, much can be done to try and reduce the risk of developing LBP, subsequent disability and work-loss.

In this chapter, the epidemiology of LBP (not including leg pain) will be presented to highlight the magnitude of this problem. Factors increase the risk of LBP, and persistent symptoms, an evidence-based perspective will then be addressed. A range of evidence including current occupational and clinical guidelines for the management of LBP will be presented, with particular focus being placed on providing practical lifestyle advice in a clinical context. It is anticipated that this advice resource will enable health care professionals to provide patients with appropriate and up-to-date information. However, it is not meant to be used as a tool for diagnosing back pain, and readers are advised to work within the scope of their professional practice. Owing to the vast literature on back pain, the following is a selective account summarising the evidence pertinent to the aims of this book.

The cost of LBP

The extensive social and health care costs linked to low back emphasise the need to intervene with effective approaches. In 1994, the Clinical Standards Advisory Group (CSAG) conducted a survey which estimated that work-loss due to back pain was about 52 million days, with 106 million being spent in benefits. Therefore, the consequences of disability are costly, although not all workers will cease work. A 4-week study of 1136 working people with back pain found that only 6% had been absent due to their symptoms (Mason, 1994). However, it is known that from those workers who take sickness absence, about 1% will go on to long-term incapacity (Waddell and Burton, 2000). Recent evidence from a series of standardised surveys completed by the Health and Safety Executive provides a more detailed indication of the prevalence of sickness absence due to back pain (HSE, 1999, 2003). Since 1995, the prevalence of self-reported work-related low back pain (LBP) has fallen (HSE, 1999), although the number of annual working days lost in 2003 (32.9 million) is substantially higher than in 1995 (18 million). Coyle and Richardson (1994) estimated the National Health Service (NHS) costs of health care for back pain in the UK in 1993 as £420 million. Taking into account the additional cost of work-loss and state benefits, the total cost of back pain in the UK was approximately £6 billion.

Epidemiological overview of LBP

In order to understand the epidemiology of LBP, it is important to first understand some common epidemiologic terms:

Incidence is the rate at which new cases of a symptom occur in a given population who were initially free of the symptoms during a specified time period.

Prevalence is the proportion of people in a defined population who have a symptom at a specific time (point prevalence), or within a stated period of time (period prevalence).

Hazards have the potential to do harm, whilst risk determinants dictate the actual probability of someone coming to harm, and are referred to as risk or protective factors.

An association means that the probability of the occurrence of one factor depends on one or more other factors, and this relationship maybe causal or non-causal.

LBP in the general population

In the UK, a cross-sectional community survey of 7699 adults, with prospective follow-up has shown LBP to have a 1-month prevalence of 39%, and a lifetime prevalence of 58% (Papageorgiou *et al.*, 1995). Such findings are comparable to surveys by Mason (1994) and Hillman *et al.* (1996), who found the lifetime prevalence to be 58–59%. Mason (1994) and Hillman *et al.* (1996) found the point and annual prevalence rates to be 14–19% and 37–39% respectively. These annual prevalence figures are supported by data from the Department of Health (DH, 1999), who established this to be 40%, the same level they reported in 1996 (DH, 1996). Young people are also known to have prevalence rates similar to those of adults with back pain (Burton *et al.*, 1996).

LBP in working populations

Attempts to consider occupational LBP as a separate set of symptoms to that experienced by the general population may be unfounded. Waddell and Burton (2000) state that LBP can be considered occupational in the sense that it is common in adults of working age and may present as an occupational health problem. Therefore, workers do get LBP and may perceive that their symptoms were caused by work (Linton and Warg, 1993), but the relationship between occupational exposure and LBP is complex and inconsistent. Several studies have demonstrated that low back disorders are particularly prevalent in certain occupations. High prevalence rates are found among agricultural workers, construction workers, carpenters, drivers, nurses, cleaners, orderlies and domestic assistants (De Beeck and Hermans, 2000). The prevalence of self-reported LBP is similar amongst sedentary and manual workers (Fahrbach and Chapman, 1990). Therefore, certain jobs may increase the risk of LBP, but when viewed overall, physical working conditions account for only a modest proportion of LBP occurring in workers (Waddell and Burton, 2000).

The course of LBP

Previous studies investigating recovery from LBP have shown that 75–90% of acute episodes presenting in General Practice improve within six weeks (Pengel *et al.*, 2003). However, although after six weeks most patients cease to consult their doctor and return to work, the majority continue to experience symptoms (Pengel *et al.*, 2003). Croft *et al.* (1998) conducted a prospective study and found that 75% of patients had persistent LBP after 1 year. This finding is supported by evidence from a recent prospective study of adults attending an osteopathic practice (Burton *et al.*, 2004). During a 4-year follow-up, symptom recurrence was reported by 78% of respondents, with half seeking further care (Burton *et al.*, 2004). Therefore, it is axiomatic that LBP is now known as a recurrent, intermittent and episodic lifetime phenomenon for the vast majority of people afflicted (Croft *et al.*, 1998; Adams *et al.*, 2002).

Lifestyle-related risk factors for LBP

The origin of LBP is complicated and mutifactorial, depending on the interrelationships between a broad range of individual and physical (environmental) risk factors. This section will consider those factors related to a patient's lifestyle that might be amenable to change. Whilst prevention of the first onset of LBP maybe unrealistic, understanding lifestyle-related risk factors could help to reduce the risk of recurrence, a concept that has been termed 'primary prevention' (Frank *et al.*, 1996).

Impact of the following individual lifestyle factors are briefly outlined for patients in Handouts 4.1 and 4.2. Talking openly with the patient regarding each lifestyle factor may help influence lifestyle modification which may in turn address some of the factors associated with LBP.

Individual risk factors

Smoking

A large number of studies have linked back pain to smoking, and based on the results of magnetic resonance imaging showing increased disc degeneration in smokers compared to non-smokers, it has been proposed that smoking can reduce blood flow to the intervertebral disc, thus impairing nutrition (Battie *et al.*, 1991).

However, smoking behaviour could be influenced by a range of demographic, psychosocial and lifestyle factors that alter the risk of back pain, but as of yet these are poorly understood. Deyo and Bass (1989) conducted a large population study, and found that people who smoked three or more packets per day were at increased risk of developing back pain than non-smokers. These results were unaffected even after allowing for exercise and obesity. Therefore, on balance, the literature suggests that there is a higher prevalence of back pain associated with smoking, although this effect is considered to be weak, and it is not clear if this is causal.

Obesity

Leboeuf-Yde (2000) conducted a systematic review of 65 studies investigating the relationship between obesity and LBP, and found that 32% of all the studies reported a statistically significant positive association between body weight and LBP. However, this association was weak, and at present there is no convincing evidence to support the popular clinical opinion that increased body weight or obesity increases the risk of LBP. Indeed, it is feasible that an individual who experiences repeated bouts of LBP may be predisposed to inactivity, thus increasing their weight.

Physical activity and sport in leisure time

Physical activity in leisure time could either protect against or increase the risk of LBP (Abenhaim *et al.*, 2000). Nourbakhsh *et al.* (2001) evaluated the effects of leisure activity on LBP, and the occurrence of symptoms was found to be significantly lower in subjects who exercised regularly. However, sedentary workload and activity was self-reported, and is not valid for studying exposure–effect relationships (Viikari-Juntari *et al.*, 1996). In contrast, studies have also reported no association between LBP and leisure activity (Rossignol *et al.*, 1993; Kuaja *et al.*, 1996; Croft *et al.*, 1999). Campell *et al.* (1996) concluded that rigorous studies do support the hypothesis that general exercise protects against LBP. A systematic review has also found that sedentary leisure activity is associated with a higher prevalence of LBP and absence in sedentary workers (Hildebrandt *et al.*, 2000).

Sporting activity could infer separate levels of risk to 'general activity' (Jacob *et al.*, 2004). A 10-year prospective study carried out by Leino (1993) found that people who took regular physical exercise has fewer back pain symptoms. Weightlifting and gymnastics have both been found to increase the risk of disc degeneration, but this is not always symptomatic (Sward *et al.*, 1991; Videman *et al.*, 1995).

Athletes in general do not experience any more back pain than non-athletes, suggesting that intense physical activity might well have a protective effect on back pain.

Despite inconsistent evidence of an influence on the risk of back pain, there are strong cardiovascular, musculoskeletal and physiological benefits from exercise, so physical activity should be promoted as beneficial to lumbar health (DH, 2004). Therefore, whilst general leisure activity is thought to be beneficial, sporting activities that involve lifting, twisting, pulling and pushing may increase risk (Vuori, 2001). Different types of exercise are also thought to have different effects on LBP. Yoga exercises are thought to increase spinal flexibility, thus reducing the risk of flexion injuries to the spine, and the incidence of LBP. Popular 'core-stability' type exercises designed to improve the endurance of specific abdominal and back muscles are more effective at reducing recurrences of LBP than doing general exercise (Hides *et al.*, 2001). Importantly the presence of LBP does not preclude the use of activity; in fact, treatment with physical activity is known to enhance physical function and mental health (Iverson *et al.*, 2003).

Physical (environmental) risk factors

Most modern lifestyles revolve around work, where exposure to physical factors can increase the risk of back pain. There is a plethora of research in this area, although researchers rarely consider the additive effect of exposure to 'occupational hazards' in leisure time. This section will broadly consider lifestyle-related environmental risks, and the term 'work' will be used to relate to meaningful activity, not just paid employment.

Sedentary work, sitting and driving

It has been postulated that sedentary work can increase the risk of back pain (Gordon, 1990; Wittink *et al.*, 1999), although this type of work has also been found to have a neutral or protective influence (Hoogendoorn *et al.*, 1999). Therefore, the evidence is not consistent, and maybe due to researchers using inadequate and noncomparable techniques to assess exposure to sedentary work (Viikari-Juntari *et al.*, 1996).

Sitting is widely regarded as a hazard of sedentary work, although this popular view no longer stands scientific scrutiny. A review by Hartvigsen *et al.* (2000) included studies published between 1985 and 1997. Only 8 out of 35 had a satisfactory experimental design, and all but one failed to find a positive association. Furthermore, all but three of the studies were cross-sectional and probably subject to the healthy worker effect (Rossignol *et al.*, 1992; Riihimaki *et al.*, 1994; Rothenbacher *et al.*, 1997). It was concluded that the literature does not support the view that sitting at work is associated with back pain. A recent review also failed to find any association between sitting and back pain (Lis *et al.*, 2007). However, when awkward postures and driving whilst sitting were separately considered, risk significantly increased for each activity. Driving in particular might also carry an increased risk of disc prolapse (Kelsey, 1975), and several authors have identified that exposure to whole body vibration (whilst driving) is linked to LBP (Hulshof and van Zanten, 1987; Pope *et al.*, 1999). This is thought to be because the dominant frequency of most vehicles is 4–6 Hz, which also happens to be the resonating frequency of the spine (Pope *et al.*, 1998). Therefore, certain sedentary occupations are thought to increase the risk of LBP, and these might well have a cumulative effect, emphasising the importance of exercise (see Handouts 4.2 and 4.3).

Manual work

Manual work is used here to incorporate manual handling, lifting, bending and twisting activities. The evidence in this area is best summarised by the UK Occupational Health Guidelines for the Management of Low Back Pain at work (Carter and Birrell, 2000). These guidelines show that there is strong evidence that physical demands (manual handling, lifting, bending, twisting) are a risk factor for the onset of LBP, but overall it appears that the size of the effect is less than that of individual and unidentified factors. These physical demands can be associated with increased reports of back symptoms, aggravation of symptoms and 'injuries'.

Psychosocial impact on lifestyle and LBP disability

Although reported pain severity and distribution are important, psychosocial factors are more strongly implicated in the transition from acute to chronic pain. These have been termed 'obstacles to recovery' (Main and Burton, 2000; Waddell and Burton, 2005), since their absence (or low level) reduce the risk of disability. Therefore, how an individual who develops back pain behaves depends on the psychosocial factors that perfuse that individuals' life, and whilst most people react normally, some will not recover. For instance, the decision to visit a GP or to take analgesics maybe perfectly understandable given that tissue damage might be associated with anxiety. In this circumstance, symptoms might well be reported, but the tendency is to recover spontaneously (Walker, 2000). Psychosocial factors and beliefs about symptoms are known to influence such care-seeking behaviour (Waddell, 1987). Therefore, the decision to seek health care depends strongly on the person's perceptions and their interpretation of the significance of their symptoms. Patients are known to have expectations about the need for diagnosis and treatment. However, the vast majority of symptoms are self-limiting and relate to a diagnosis of non-specific LBP, and do not require treatment to recover. So, expectations about medical intervention and back pain are shaped by life experiences and interactions. The role of medical professionals is to identify irrational beliefs, for example, the need for lengthy treatment in which the patient plays a 'passive role', in order to try and prevent the development of chronic pain, this being termed 'secondary prevention'.

Some individuals will not seek health care, and there is no evidence that the pain intensity of patients reporting back pain is greater than that of individuals who manage the problem themselves (Waddell, 1999). However, a small minority of patients will not recover, becoming disabled and taking prolonged absence from work. These are also examples of pain behaviour, but are maladaptive and develop as a consequence of psychosocial factors that obstruct recovery (Marhold, 2002). In these patients the pain, which becomes prolonged, seems to be disassociated from tissue damage (Jones *et al.*, 2003). At this point it is useful to make the distinction between pain and disability, as not everyone who has recurrent or persistent back pain becomes disabled. Pain is clearly a symptom, and disability relates to some degree of restricted activity (WHO, 2001). But pain is more than an aversive sensation, having cognitive and behavioural dimensions. So, in the presence of pain, psychosocial (clinical and occupational) factors will influence how an individual thinks, and need to be addressed because they have shown to predict lifestyle decisions (e.g. sickness absence).

Psychological distress – for example, depressive symptoms and low mood are a risk factor for the development of disability (Pincus *et al.*, 2002). This might relate to other factors, for example, social isolation, lack of support.

Fear avoidance beliefs – the cognitive model of fear of movement/(re)injury, proposes that individuals who believe that activity will aggravate their pain will expect/fear more pain if they are active (Vlaeyen and Crombez, 1999). This is thought to play an integral part in the avoidance of activity and the transition from acute back pain to disability (Crombez *et al.*, 1999). Overcoming fear avoidance beliefs is a key message from useful patient handouts such as 'The Back Book' (Burton *et al.*, 1999), and has shown to help improve beliefs amongst patients and reduce disability (Burton *et al.*, 1999).

Job satisfaction – if an individual is dissatisfied with this aspect of their life they are more likely to take time off from work with back pain (Waddell and Burton, 2001). The influence of such 'psychosocial aspect of work' maybe difficult to modify.

Social support – there is some evidence that a lifestyle with high levels of social support (e.g. at work) can help to prevent disability (Morken *et al.*, 2003). Health care providers are an attractive form of support, and should work with patients to direct them to (and follow-up) their engagement with community or work-related services to promote coping strategies. This should improve their ability to cope.

Lifestyle management in the treatment of LBP

The main problem with back pain is not that symptoms occur, but that some individuals make lifestyle decisions that lead to compromised quality of life and disability. Failure to recover is known to partly relate to the traditional belief that bed rest is beneficial, and that since pain hurts, you should rest until it goes away (Deyo, 1998). These beliefs are based on the notion that pain is proportional to damage, although with non-specific back pain there is little evidence of damage, and it is important that patients understand that hurt does equal harm. Clinical (Royal College of General Practitioners [RCGP], 1999) and occupational (Carter and Birrell, 2000) health guidelines have reviewed the evidence to inform health professionals: there is strong evidence that advice to continue ordinary activities of daily living as normally as possible despite pain can give equivalent or faster recovery from acute symptoms, and fewer recurrences and work-loss over the following year than traditional advice to rest (RCGP, 1999). There is also moderate evidence that advice to continue ordinary activities of daily living can be supplemented by educational interventions designed to overcome fear avoidance beliefs and encourage patients to take responsibility for their own self-care. Specific exercises do not produce clinically significant improvements in acute LBP.

Contrary to popular belief, there is strong evidence that most workers with back pain are able to continue working or return to work within a few days or weeks, even if they still have some symptoms, and they do not need to wait until they are pain free (Carter and Birrell, 2000). Indeed, advice to continue activities as normally as possible, in principle, applies equally to work. However, the belief that returning to work with residual symptoms will increase the risk of re-injury is commonplace (Waddell and Burton, 2001). Epidemiological studies have conclusively shown that back pain can persist for several months, and symptom recurrence is commonplace (Coste *et al.*, 1994; Croft *et al.*, 1998). So, if no workers returned to work until they were symptom free, only a minority would ever return to work (Carter and Birrell, 2000). Workers with symptoms are also known to both continue working without taking absence, or return to work with symptoms (Carey *et al.*, 2000). Therefore, remaining at work or returning to work with symptoms is not detrimental and will reduce recurrences and sickness absence over the next year (Waddell *et al.*, 1997; Abenhaim *et al.*, 2000). There is moderate evidence that the temporary provision of lighter or modified duties can facilitate return to normal work and reduce absence (Krause *et al.*, 1998).

Conclusion

Back pain is a normal consequence of life for many people, and the decisions that we make can have an impact on both the risk of developing back pain, and its recovery. Care-seeking behaviour, work absence and the development of disability following backpain are driven by our beliefs, which are in turn formed through life exposure. This chapter, whilst only glimpsing at the affect of lifestyle on back pain, offers evidence-based advice to practitioners who may come in contact with patients. Simply providing useful practical messages about how to reduce the risk of recurrence and optimise recovery could prove invaluable to patients, helping to eradicate the myths and irrational beliefs that are held about back pain, which exert such a powerful influence on our lives.

References

Abenhaim, L., Rossignol, M., Valat, J. P. *et al.* (2000). The role of activity in the therapeutic management of back pain: report of the international Paris task force on back pain. *Spine*, 25(4): 1S–31S.

Adams, M., Bogduk, N., Burton, K. and Dolan, P. (2002). *The Biomechanics of Back Pain*. Edinburgh, Churchill Livingstone.

Battie, M. C., Videman, T., Gill, K., Moneta, G. B., Nyman, R., *et al.* (1991). Smoking and lumbar intervertebral disc degeneration: an MRI study of identical twins. *Spine*, 16: 1015–1021.

Burton, A. K., Clark, R. D., McCluune, T. D., Tillotson, K. M. (1996). The natural history of low back pain in adolescents. *Spine*, 21(20): 2323–2328.

Burton, A. K., McClune, T. D., Clarke, R. D. and Main, C. J. (2004). Long term follow-up of patients with low back pain attending manipulative care: outcomes and predictors. *Manual Therapy*, 9(1): 30–35.

Burton, A. K., Waddell, G., Tillotson, K. M. and Summerton, N. (1999). Information and advice to patients with back pain can have a positive effect. A randomised controlled trial of a novel educational booklet in primary care. *Spine*, 24(23): 2484–2491.

Campell, M., Nordin, N. and Weiser, S. (1996). Physical exercise and low back pain. *Scandinavian Journal of Medicine, Science & Sports*, 6(2): 63–72.

Carey, T. S., Garrett, J. and Jackman, A. (2000). Beyond the good prognosis: examination of an inception cohort of patients with chronic low back pain. *Spine*, 25: 2210–2219.

Carter, J. T. and Birrell, L. N. (2000). *Occupational Health Guidelines for the Management of Low Back Pain at Work – Principal Recommendations*. London, Faculty of Occupational Medicine.

Coste, J., Delecoeuillerie, G., Cohen de Lara, A., Le Parc, J. M. and Paolaggi, J. B. (1994). Clinical course and prognostic factors in acute low back pain: an inception cohort study in primary care practice. *British Medical Journal*, 308(6928): 577–580.

Coyle, D. and Richardson, G. (1994). The cost of back pain. In *Clinical Standards Advisory Group. Epidemiology Review: The Epidemiology and Cost of Back Pain*. London, HMSO.

Croft, P. R., Macfarlene G. J., Papageorgiou, A. C., Thomas, E. and Silman, A. J. (1998). Outcome of low back pain in general practice: a prospective study. *British Medical Journal*, 316: 1356–1359.

Croft, P., Papageorgiou, A. C., Thomas, E., Macfarlane, G. J. and Silman, A. J. (1999). Short term physical risk factors for new episodes of low back pain. Prospective evidence from the South Manchester back pain study. *Spine*, 24(15): 1556–1561.

Crombez, G., Vlaeyen, J. W., Heuts, P. H. G. and Lysens, R. (1999). Pain related fear is more disabling than pain itself: evidence on the role of pain related fear in chronic back pain disability. *Pain*, 80: 329–339.

De Beeck, R. O. and Hermans, V. (2000). Research on Work Related Low Back Disorders. Report of the European Agency for Safety and Health at Work. Belgium, Institute for Occupational Safety and Health, 3–70.

Deyo, R. A. and Bass, J. E. (1989). Lifestyle and low-back pain: The influence of smoking and obesity. *Spine*, 14(5): 501–506.

Deyo, R. A. (1998). Low back pain. *Scientific American*, 279: 53.

DH (1996). *The Prevalence of Back Pain in Great Britain*. London, Office of National Statistics, 1–15.

DH (1999). The prevalence of back pain in Great Britain in 1998. *A Report on Research for the Department of Health Using the ONS Omnibus Survey*. London, HMSO.

DH (2004). *At Least Five a Week. Physical Activity and Musculoskeletal Health*. P. A. Department of Health, Health Improvement and Prevention, 53–48.

Fahrbach, P. A. and Chapman, L. J. (1990). VDT work duration and musculoskeletal discomfort. *AAOHN Journal*, 38(1): 32–36.

Frank, J. W., Kerr, M. S., Brooker, A. S. *et al.* (1996). Disability resulting from occupational low back pain part 1: what do we know about primary prevention? A review of the scientific evidence on prevention before disability begins. *Spine*, 21: 2908–2917.

Gordon, G. A. (1990). A molecular basis for low back pain in Western industrialised cultures. *Medical Hypotheses*, 33: 251–256.

Hartvigsen, J., Leboeuf-Yde, C., Lings, S., Corder, E. H. (2000). Is sitting-while-at-work associated with low back pain? A systematic, critical literature review. *Scandinavian Journal of Public Health*, 28(3): 230–239.

Hides, J. A., Jull, G. A. and Richardson, C. A. (2001). Long term effects of specific stabilising exercises for first episode low back pain. *Spine*, 26(11): E243–E248.

Hildebrandt, V. H., Bongers, P. M., Dull, J., van Dijk, F. J. and Kemper, H. C. (2000). The relationship between leisure time, physical activities and musculoskeletal symptoms and disability in worker populations. *International Archives of Occupational and Environmental Health*, 73(8): 507–518.

Hillman, M., Wright, A., Rajaratnam, G., Tennant, A., Chamberlain, M. A. (1996). Prevalence of low back pain in the community: implications for service provision in Bradford UK. *J Epidemiol Community Health*, 50: 347–352.

Hoogendoorn, W. E., Poppel, M. N. M. and Bongers, P. M. (1999). Physical load during work and leisure time as risk factors for back pain. *Scandinavian Journal of Work and Environmental Health*, 25: 387–403.

HSE (1999). *The Costs to Britain of Work Place Accidents and Work Related Ill Health in 1995/1996*. Norwich, HMSO.

HSE (2003). *Self Reported Work-Related Illness 2001/02: Results of a Household Survey*. Norwich, HMSO.

Hulshof, C. and van Zanten, B. V. (1987). Whole body vibration and low back pain. A review of epidemiologic studies. *Internal Archives of Occupational and Environmental Health*, 59: 205–220.

Iverson, M. D. E., Fossel, A. H. and Katz, J. N. (2003). Enhancing function in older adults with chronic low back pain: a pilot study of endurance training. *Archives of Physical Medicine and Rehabilitation*, 84: 1324–1331.

Jacob, T., Baras, A., Zeev, A. and Epstein, L. (2004). Physical activities and low back pain: a community based study. *Medicine and Science in Sports and Exercise*, 36(1): 9–15.

Jones, J. R., Huxtable, C. S., Hodgson, J. and Price, M. J. (eds) (2003). *Self Reported Work Related Illness in 2001/2002: Results from a Household Survey*. HSE Books, Sudbury.

Kelsey, J. L. (1975). An epidemiological study of the relationship between occupations and acute herniated lumbar intervertebral discs. *International Journal of Epidemiology*, 4: 197–204.

Krause, N., Dasinger, L. K. and Neuhauser, F. (1998). Modified work and return to work: a review of the literature. *Journal of Occupational Rehabilitation*, 8: 113–139.

Kuaja, U. M., Taimela, S. and Viljanen, T. (1996). Physical loading and performance as predictors of back pain in healthy adults: a 5 year prospective study. *Journal of Applied Physiology*, 73: 452–458.

Leboeuf-Yde, C., (2000). Body weight and low back pain: A systematic literature review of 56 journal articles reporting on 65 epidemiologic studies. *Spine*, 25(2): 226.

Leino, P. I., (1993). Does leisure time physical activity prevent low back disorders? A prospective study of metal industry employees. *Spine*, 18(7): 863–871.

Linton, S. J. and Warg, L. E. (1993). Attributions (beliefs) and job satisfaction associated with back pain in an industrial setting. *Perceptual Motor Skills*, 76(1): 51–62.

Lis, A. M., Black, K. M., Korn, H. and Nordin, M. (2007). Association between sitting and occupational LBP. *European Spine Journal*, 16: 283–298.

Main, C. J. and Burton, A. K. (2000). Economic and occupational influences on pain and disability. In Main, C. J. and Spanswick, C. C. (eds) *Pain Managament: An Interdisciplinary Approach*. Edinburgh, Churchill Livingstone, 63–87.

Marhold, C. (2002). Musculoskeletal pain and return to work. A cognitive-behavioral perspective. Acta Universitatis Upsaliensis. *Comprehensive Summaries of Uppsala Dissertations from the Faculty of Social Sciences*, 113, p. 78.

Mason, V. (1994). *The Prevalence of Back Pain in Great Britain*. London, Office of Population Censuses and Surveys Social Survey Division.

Morken, T., Riise, T., Moen, B. *et al.* (2003). Low back pain and widespread pain predicts sickness absence among industrial workers. *BMC Musculoskeletal Disorders*, 4(21): 1–8.

New Zealand Guidelines Group (2003). *New Zealand Acute Low Back Pain Guide*. Wellington, New Zealand.

Nourbakhsh, M. R., Moussavi, S. J. and Salavati, M. (2001). Effects of lifestyle and work-related physical activity on the degree of lumbar lordosis and chronic low back pain in a Middle East population. *Journal of Spinal Disorders*, 14: 283–292.

Papageorgiou, A. C., Croft, P. R. and Ferry, S. (1995). Estimating the prevalence of low back pain in the general population: evidence from the South Manchester back pain survey. *Spine*, 20: 1889–1894.

Pengel, L. H. M., Herbert, R. D., Maher, C. G. and Refshauge, K. M. (2003). Acute low back pain: systematic review of its prognosis. *British Medical Journal*, 327(9): 1–5.

Pincus, T., Burton, A. K., Vogel, S. and Field, A. P. (2002). A systematic review of psychological factors as predictors of chronicity/disability in prospective cohorts of low back pain. *Spine*, 27(5): 109–120.

Pope, M. H., Magnusson, M. and Wilder, D. G. (1998). Kappa delta award. Low back pain and whole body vibration. *Clinical Orthopaedics*, 354: 241–248.

Pope, M. H., Wilder, D. G. and Magnusson, M. L. (1999). A review of studies on seated whole body vibration and low back pain. *Mechanical Engineering*, 213(6): 435–446.

RCGP (1999). *Clinical Guidelines for the Management of Low Back Pain*. London, Royal College of General Practitioners.

Riihimaki, H., Vikari-Juntura, E., Moneta, G., Kuha, J., Videman, T. and Tola, S. (1994). Incidence of sciatic pain among men in machine operating, dynamic physical work, and sedentary work. *Spine*, 19: 138–142.

Rossignol, M., Lortie, M. and Ledoux, E. (1993). Comparison of spinal health indicators in predicting spinal status in a 1 year longitudinal study. *Spine*, 18: 54–60.

Rossignol, M., Suissa, S. and Abenhaim, L. (1992). Working disability due to occupational back pain: three year follow up of 2,300 compensated workers in Quebec. *Journal of Occupational Medicine*, 30: 502–505.

Rothenbacher, D., Brenner, H., Arndt, V., Fraisse, E., Zschenderlein, B. and Fliedner, T. M. (1997). Disorders of the back and spine in construction workers. Prevalence and prognostic value for disability. *Spine*, 22: 1481–1486.

Sward, L., Hellstrom, M., Jacobsson, B., Nyman, R. and Peterson, L. (1991). Disc degeneration and associated abnormalities of the spine in elite gymnasts. A magnetic resonance imaging study. *Spine*, 16(4): 437–443.

Van Tulder, M., Malmivaara, A. and Esmail, R. K., B. (2000). Exercise therapy for low back pain. A systematic review within the framework of the cochrane collaboration back review group. *Spine*, 25(21): 2784–2796.

Videmann, T. and Battie, M. C. (1999). The influence of occupation on lumbar degeneration. *Spine*, 24: 1164–1168.

Viikari-Juntari, E., Rauas, S., Martikainen, R. *et al.* (1996). Validity of self reported physical work load in epidemiologic studies on musculoskeletal disorders. *Scandinavian Journal of Work and Environmental Health*, 22(4): 251–259.

Vlaeyen, J. W. S. and Crombez, G. (1999). Fear of movement (re)injury and pain disability in chronic low back pain patients. *Manual Therapy*, 4(4): 187–195.

Vuori, E. M. (2001). Dose–response of physical activity and low back pain, osteoarthritis and osteoporosis. *Medicine and Science in Sports and Exercise*, 9: 1451–1458.

Waddell, G. (1987). A new clinical model for the treatment of low back pain. *Spine*, 7: 632–644.

Waddell, G. (1999). *The Back Pain Revolution*. Edinburgh, Churchill Livingstone.

Waddell, G. and Burton, A. K. (2000). *Occupational Health Guidelines for the Management of Low Back Pain at Work-Evidence Review*. London, Faculty of Occupational Medicine.

Waddell, G. and Burton, A. K. (2001). Occupational health guidelines for the management of low back pain at work: evidence review. *Occupational Medicine*, 51(2): 124–135.

Waddell, G. and Burton, A. K. (2005). *Concepts of Rehabilitation for the Management of Common Health Problems*. London, Department for Work and Pensions.

Waddell, G., Feder, G. and Lewis, M. (1997). Systematic reviews of bed rest and advice to stay active for acute low back pain. *British Journal of General Practice*, 47: 647–652.

Walker, B. F. (2000). The prevalence of low back pain: a systematic review of the literature from 1966 to 1998. *Journal of Spinal Disorders*, 13(3): 205–217.

WHO (2001). International Classification of Functioning, Disability and Health. Geneva, World Health Organisation.

Wittink, H., Michel, T. H., Wagner, A., Sukiennik, A. and Rogers, W. (1999). Deconditioning in patients with chronic low back pain: fact or fiction? *Spine*, 25(17): 2221–2228.

Useful patient resources

The Back Book: www.tsoshop.co.uk/bookstore.asp?FO=1159966&Action=Book&ProductID=0117029491.

Back care leaflets: www.backpain.org/pages/e_pages/exercise.php

Backcare: www.backcare.org.uk

All of the following handouts and advice boxes can be found as individual pdfs on the website at www.blackwellpublishing.com/thew

Advice box 4.1 Advice – 'based on the epidemiology' (Handout 4.1)

- Back pain is likely to be experienced by the majority of people during their life, and for many this will become a recurrent problem.
- Patients should not worry about symptoms, because they are a normal consequence of life, similar to getting grey hair.
- Do not necessarily be concerned if a young person presents with back pain, they have a similar prevalence to adults.
- Certain jobs are associated with an increased prevalence of back pain, but for many individuals symptoms at work are purely coincidental. So, beliefs about the hazardous effects of many jobs are misplaced, and patients should not seek to change jobs because of back pain.
- It is normal to have 'good' and 'bad days' during recovery, and patients should not be concerned if they suddenly experience a 'bad day'.

Advice box 4.2 Advice – 'modifying individual risk factors' (Handout 4.1)

- Smoking is not good for health, and although the evidence is equivocal, it may increase the risk of back pain. Patients should be counselled to stop smoking.
- Obesity is weakly associated with back pain, and does not appear to increase the risk of back pain.
- Advice to lose weight in an effort to reduce the risk of future or current symptoms is not supported by evidence. But, since activity might have a protective effect, if advice is to be offered, it should focus on increasing activity, not dieting.
- Physical activity should be encouraged to maintain and improve lumbar health – there is certainly no evidence of a detrimental effect. Being active with back pain does have a proven beneficial effect (see Handout 4.2).

Advice box 4.3 Advice – 'modifying environmental risk factors' (Handout 4.1)

- A sedentary lifestyle does not seem to cause back pain, and may actually reduce risk. Patients should be advised that 'office work' is likely to be quite good for their back, and should not be blamed for their symptoms.
- Sitting on its own is not related to back pain, but awkward postures or driving whilst sitting do seem to increase risk. Regular breaks from sitting are advisable.
- Professionals should not focus on helping patients to achieve a 'correct' sitting posture; current evidence does not support the view of a good or bad posture, and patients should sit in whatever posture is comfortable.
- There is strong evidence that physical demands at work can cause recurrent attacks of back pain, although these will not necessarily have caused the initial onset of symptoms.

Advice box 4.4 Advice – 'related to psychosocial influences on lifestyle'

- Care-seeking is a coping response, so all patients who present to a health professional are potentially vulnerable to disability.
- Health professionals should identify the concerns/expectations of their patients (e.g. need for diagnosis and treatment), and educational material can be used to accurately inform them (Handout 4.2).
- Attempts should be made to reassure patients and modify irrational beliefs about back pain, for example, moving will make symptoms worse and cause further damage. There is evidence that this type of educational input using 'the back book' can modify beliefs (Burton *et al.*, 1999).
- Clinical and occupational psychosocial factors should be screened at consultation to determine risk of disability (Carter and Birrell, 2000; New Zealand Guidelines Group, 2003).

Advice box 4.5 Advice – 'management of back pain' (Handout 4.2)

- Patients who present with acute back pain should be discouraged from rest. Rather, advice to continue normal activities of daily living will help to increase the rate of recovery.
- Whilst specific exercises have not shown to produce 'statistically significant' improvements, theoretically they are beneficial, but should not be used as a replacement for 'general activity'.
- Patients should be advised to return to work even if they have symptoms, and perhaps undertake modified work duties.
- The risk of disability increases the longer that a patient is off work, so returning to work or modified work as soon as possible is the key.

Handout 4.1 Facts about back pain

The problem. Back pain is a common problem that affects most of us at some point in our lives, just like getting grey hair!

Back pain is not usually due to any serious problem.

Lots of people who get back pain experience repeated episodes throughout their life, and this is very common.

Many people will experience back pain at work, but this does not mean that work caused the symptoms. In fact, getting back pain at work might be a coincidence, for example, you were going to get it anyway.

Reducing the risk of back pain. Smoking is not good for your health, and is thought to interfere with the nutrition supply to the disc. Smoking might increase your risk of back pain!

Being overweight is not good for health, and has found to be related to back pain. In order to lose weight (and perhaps reduce your risk of back pain), regular physical activity comes highly recommended.

Being physically active is thought to be good for spinal health, and will give you stronger muscles and bones and make you feel good. Regular walking, cycling or swimming are all beneficial.

Sitting too much is not thought to increase the risk of back pain, although sitting in a constrained or awkward position, and driving for long periods of time is thought to increase risk. Backcare offers practical advice on how best to reduce risk when driving (http://www.backpain.org/pdfs/backcare-for-drivers.pdf).

Manual work probably aggravates symptoms in people who already have back pain, but is not thought to cause symptoms in the first place. So, it is important to adopt a correct lifting technique and to follow manual handling guidelines that are provided, if manual work relates to your job.

Despite the above measures, reducing the risk of back pain is difficult, so do not be surprised if you still experience back pain. The key issue is to be positive and to get active! (see Handout 4.2).

Handout 4.2 Management of back pain

Diagnosis and treatment. Back pain is rarely due to any serious disease and does not usually require treatment to get better. But, if your symptoms appear to be getting worse rather than better (over several weeks), for example, you feel unwell, have difficulty passing urine, have numbness around your back passage/genitals, or have numbness/pins and needles or weakness in both legs, you should see a doctor straight away.

Special investigations such as X-rays or MRI scans cannot normally determine the source of the pain, and often show normal age-related changes.

So, if you have back pain do not worry, it is very common, and there are plenty of things that you can do to help yourself.

Activity. Patients who resume normal activities, even if they still have some pain, are known to recover more quickly than patients who rest. In fact, resting for more than several days will actually slow your recovery, causing muscles to weaken and joints to stiffen.

Exercise. Walking, cycling or swimming for 20–30 minutes every day are all good exercises that will help you to recover from your episode of back pain more quickly than if you do not exercise. You can also try pilates, yoga or simple mobility exercises (see Handout 4.3).

Pain control. Being active and moving is perhaps the best form of pain control. You may also take paracetamol or soluble aspirin which are the simplest and safest pain killers. Or, you could use a bag of ice wrapped in a towel, a hot water bottle, a bath or a shower.

Work. Generally speaking, unless your job involves heavy lifting, you should try and return to work as soon as possible, even with symptoms. This is known to improve your rate of recovery. You could also request your employer to help provide modified activities at first.

Handout 4.3 Exercise for a better back

Spinal mobility exercises – perform daily. These exercises should be carried out slowly and deliberately. If you have pain when you perform any of them, limit the particular exercise movement so that you are comfortable. If you feel pain when you start any movement, then it should not be carried out.

Please note: These exercises can only offer general advice, since it is not possible to recommend specific exercises for your pain without having seen you. You need to decide which exercises are most appropriate for your needs. We recommend you check with your GP or chartered physiotherapist before taking up a new programme.

Source: Adapted and reproduced with kind permission from BackCare. www.backcare.org.uk Helpline: 0845 130 2704

Further exercises are available in the *Active BackCare* booklet.

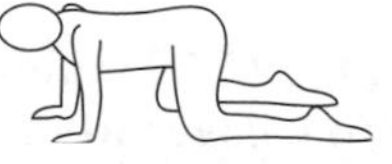

Starting position for all exercises is on all fours. Hands should be placed shoulder width apart, arms and thighs vertical. Use an exercise mat if you have one.

Arch the back, at the same time, look down at the floor. Then lower the stomach towards the floor, hollowing the back and at the same time look up to the ceiling. (if you are pregnant you should not do the second part of this exercise hollowing your back, instead keep your back straight)

Repeat 10 times.

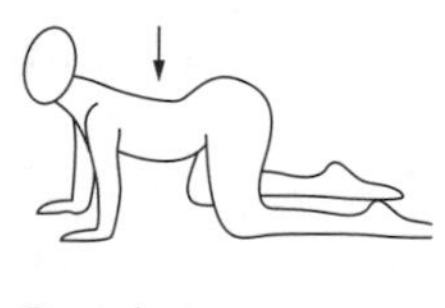

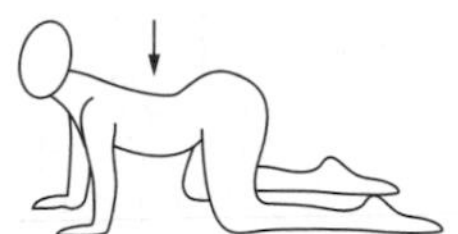

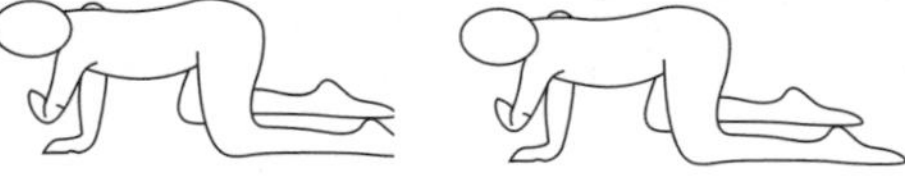

Slowly walk the hands around to the right, back to the starting position then around to the left.

Repeat 5–10 times.

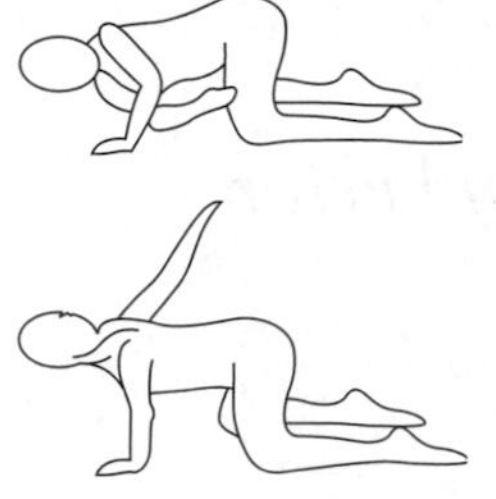

Raise one hand off the floor, reach underneath your body as far as you can.

On the return, swing the arm out to the side as far as you can, then return to the starting position.

Follow the moving hand with the eyes. Repeat with the other arm.

Repeat 5–10 times.

Draw alternate knees to the opposite elbow.

Repeat 10 times.

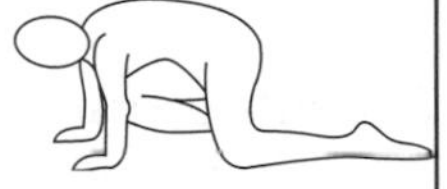

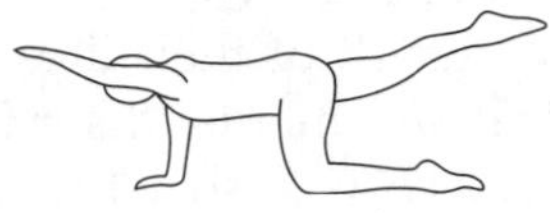

Stretch one arm forward in front, at the same time stretching the opposite leg out behind.

Repeat 10 times

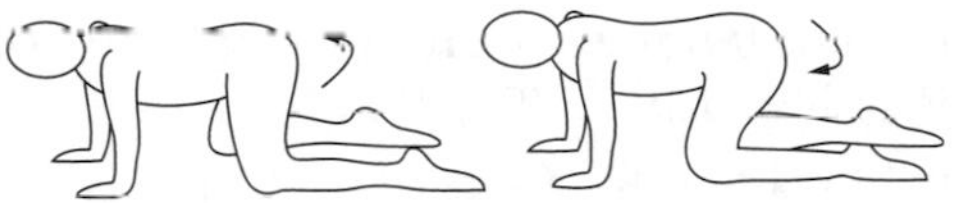

Swing the seat from side to side in a controlled manner.

Repeat 10 times.

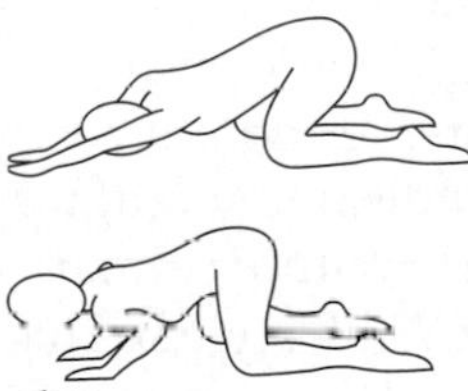

Sit back on your haunches. Lower the body forward and down so that the nose goes as close to the ground as comfortably possible. Move forward, running your nose along the ground as far as you can go before coming upright and repeating.

Repeat 10 times.

5. *Energy for Life*

Miranda Thew and Sue Pemberton

Introduction

Most people will experience a lack of energy in their lives whether as a consequence of illness or as a result of their lifestyles. Indeed, experts consider that most physical and mental disorders involve a degree of fatigue (Sharpe, 2006). The costs to society from all fatigue cases are substantial, mainly due to the amount of working days lost (McCrone *et al.*, 2003). A small but significant number of people are diagnosed with chronic fatigue syndrome (CFS)/myalgic encephalomyelitis (ME) (Wessley *et al.*, 1998; Ranjith, 2005) which can lead to severe dysfunction (Skapinakis *et al.*, 2003), and which requires expert interventions provided by specialists trained in cognitive behavioural therapy and/or graded exercise (NICE, 2007). There is already comprehensive literature and resources that support interventions with severe chronic fatigue (Chalder *et al.*, 1993; Cox, 2000). However, this specialist level of intervention is costly and largely available for those with significantly disabling fatigue symptoms.

There are opportunities particularly within primary care, to guide practitioners in providing self-help and lifestyle strategies to address wider fatigue and tiredness problems (Wearden and Chew-Graham, 2006). This chapter draws on evidence and strategies that appear to work with the more chronic and debilitating fatigue problems and applies it to more-prevalent, less-severe fatigue, which most health and social care professionals are inevitably going to encounter within their clinical practice.

Lifestyle factors are a significant causal factor for fatigue and psychological distress (Bultmann *et al.*, 2002a). Lifestyle issues such as overactive busy lives or 'action-proneness' (Van Houdenhovea *et al.*, 2001), poor sleep (Samaha *et al.*, 2007), alcohol and lack of exercise (Samaha *et al.*, 2007), being overweight with unbalanced diets (Resnick *et al.*, 2006) or looking after young children (Troy, 1999) can result in fatigue. Promising results in reducing fatigue have been found from lifestyle management programmes (Ward and Winters, 2003; McDermott *et al.*, 2004; Rossler *et al.*, 2004; Carmack Taylor *et al.*, 2007).

Therefore, lifestyle modification should be at the heart of therapeutic interventions in fatigue. By understanding the factors that may be inhibiting energy production and causing energy depletion and by adapting the occupations of daily life. The level of fatigue experienced may reduce and as a consequence, quality of life improve.

Lifestyle management for fatigue symptoms

Fatigue is a common complaint in the general adult population (Kroenke *et al.*, 1988; Bultmann *et al.*, 2005; Ranjith, 2005), which can lead to high consultation rates particularly within primary care (Hickie *et al.*, 1996; Wessley *et al.*, 1997; Haines *et al.*, 2005). Women are more likely to complain of medically unexplained fatigue than men, and significant fatigue problems are not commonly diagnosed within children or the older people (Gallagher *et al.*, 2004; Haines *et al.*, 2005). Medically unexplained fatigue can be severely disabling, particularly when correlated with psychiatric co-morbidity (Skapinakis *et al.*, 2003). Despite this, there is limited evidence of effective pharmacological, supplemental or complementary/ alternative treatments (Whiting *et al.*, 2001; NICE, 2007).

The fatigue management for primary fatigue states, such as CFS, are best treated within specialist treatment centres (DH, 2002; NICE, 2007). Although the interventions at the specialist centres are recommended to be provided by appropriately trained professionals (NICE, 2007), the lifestyle elements are largely the same as the lifestyle programmes for cardiac rehabilitation, multiple sclerosis and chronic pain. There are a number of fatigue management programmes within primary and secondary care settings demonstrating benefits, including in-patient settings for severe CFS (Cox, 1999).

Fatigue is a particularly troublesome symptom in a variety of diseases, such as cancer (Hann *et al.*, 1999; Portenoy and Itri, 1999, Loge *et al.*, 2000; Scwartz *et al.*, 2000; Curt, 2002), multiple sclerosis (Fisk *et al.*, 1994; Mathiowetz *et al.*, 2001) and cardiac problems (Puetz *et al.*, 2006), and following a stroke (Ingles *et al.*, 1999). Interventions to counteract secondary fatigue symptoms are towards encouraging self-help in aspects of lifestyle factors influencing energy balance, that is, energy output and consumption. For example, Portenoy and

Itri (1999) recommend 'patient education, stress management, modify activity and rest patterns' (p. 5) for cancer management.

Common sense and common practice

There are also 'common sense guidelines' for 'energy conservation' which is not concerned with resting *per se*, but in managing existing energy to enjoy life; in the case of managing cancer-related fatigue (CRF) these are described as

> "Energy conservation is the deliberate, planned management of an individual's personal energy resources to prevent their depletion. The objective of energy conservation is to balance rest and activity during times of high fatigue so that valued activities and goals can be maintained. Taking additional rest periods is one energy-conservation strategy. Other strategies include priority setting, delegation, pacing oneself, and planning high-energy activities at times of peak energy."
>
> (Barsevick *et al.*, 2004, p. 1303)

This common sense strategy can be expanded on in cases where pacing and priority setting may be insufficient, for example, driving if a meaningful and important life occupation may only be achieved by grading all the various components involved in driving, grading activity is much more than pacing alone (Cox, 2000; Leeds and West Yorkshire CFS Service, 2006). In other debilitating conditions, such as multiple sclerosis, fatigue symptoms are commonly ameliorated via lifestyle programmes (Ward and Winters, 2003; Roessler *et al.*, 2004).

In delivering the lifestyle management advice, the most common strategy is to apply the advice within a cognitive behavioural structure, which is the most effective form of intervention with CFS cases (Sharpe, 1998; NICE, 2007). Although, there is some evidence that cognitive behavioural therapy (CBT) is not superior to general life counselling (Ridsdale *et al.*, 2001). Others studies report poor outcomes in using a psychological approach to treat chronic fatigue, suggesting there is resistance to accepting the therapeutic rationale (Bentall *et al.*, 2002). It is, therefore, important that the health care professionals have an empathic therapeutic approach to encourage change in lifestyle factors influencing fatigue. It may be useful to refer to Chapter 1 creating the opportunity to change to encourage individuals to follow strategies that are described and advocated below.

Lifestyle management principles

General advice for managing significant symptoms of fatigue should be available within the primary care setting and should not wait until a diagnosis of primary fatigue disorder has been confirmed (NICE, 2007). The important factors within an initial fatigue management approach should include managing sleep, analyzing and supporting a healthy occupational balance including rest and relaxation and the importance of a well-balanced diet. By using time-use or activity diaries (see Handout 5.1 – inspired by Chalder, 1999) it may be possible to pick on fundamental lifestyle issues that could be contributing to fatigue. Sleep, for example, could be lacking or disturbed due to children waking in the night. Likewise, an inadequate diet that lacks essential nutrients to sustain energy may well be contributing to fatigue problems. This could be particularly so in cases of cancer where chemotherapy is causing nausea. The other chapters of this book may be used to support some of these lifestyle issues to address fatigue.

Graded exercise to improve fatigue

There is some evidence of the benefits to people with fatigue problems from graded exercise programmes (Fulcher and White, 2000; Clark and White, 2005; Moss-Morris *et al.*, 2005). Graded exercise involves exercise 'prescription', adapted to the patient's current capacity. Initial exercises can be brief and after negotiation are gradually increased either in intensity, speed or time, dependent on the extent of any after-effects (i.e. increased pain and fatigue). There appears to be no detrimental effects physiologically for people with fatigue to engage in graded exercise programmes (Edmonds *et al.*, 2004); however, those with a diagnosis of CFS complain of worsening fatigue symptoms if their exercise programme is beyond their subjected capacity (Clapp *et al.*, 1999; De Becker *et al.*, 2000), this appears unrelated to anxiety about exercise (Gallagher *et al.*, 2005) or fear of pain (Nijs *et al.*, 2004). It is therefore relevant that graded exercise with people with a diagnosis of CFS/ME should be supervised by adequately trained professionals (NICE, 2007). In terms of increasing fitness and gaining the benefits of exercise (such as a reduction in fatigue), the exercise can be incrementally reintroduced into the lives of recovering adults, for example, in cases of heart attack (Puetz *et al.*, 2006) or cancer (McNeely *et al.*, 2006). Individuals with multiple sclerosis improve subjective fatigue post-aerobic exercise (Surakka *et al.*, 2004), although only in women and not men.

Graded exercise has been seen to decrease the likelihood of people taking exaggerated rest in response to their fatigue symptoms, which could lead to de-conditioning (Clark and White, 2005). Fulcher and White (2002) found that physical de-conditioning can maintain disability in people with significant fatigue problems. Moss-Morris *et al.* (2005) conclude that graded exercise is also seen to improve psychological symptoms, despite not necessarily increasing aerobic fitness, suggesting that the focus on exercise rather than symptoms can have positive benefits for well-being. A graded exercise approach can be achieved by using an exercise or sport as the focus for the activity that is to be graded within the grading and pacing plan (stage 3) detailed below.

Four stages of lifestyle management for fatigue

Fatigue is a multi-factorial problem. Achieving lifestyle change is difficult if an individual cannot appreciate how one element can affect a multitude of symptoms. Therefore, the health care professional plays a key role in helping the person to make connections between fatigue and its relationship to other factors. Also improving energy levels is a progressive process requiring constant application. By using a gradual, staged approach to fatigue management, there can be increased compliance and longer-lasting effects from interventions (Cox, 1999; Von Korff and Tiemens, 2000). Each of these stages is illustrated below but essentially are

Stage one: Effective management of fatigue requires a supportive and collaborative relationship with the client (NICE, 2007). Fatigue as a symptom is difficult to appreciate in another person, and often it can appear to be an insignificant problem. Scenarios can help explain how fatigue affects people, and in turn help individuals to appreciate how their subjective behaviours in response to fatigue is possibly increasing the problem.

Stage two: By specifically identifying the different variables that are impacting upon energy via completion of a energy/time use diary (Handout 5.1), overall personal lifestyle can be revealed. This encourages people to analyse their life activities and how they are performing them including identifying base lines. Other life factors such as relationships can have a draining or energising effect and are also important to consider (Handout 5.2).

Stage three: This involves suggesting strategies that can adapt the way in which they engage with the daily occupations or routines of life, that is, grading and pacing, or how to deal with life draining factors, such as using relaxation to combat stress.

Stage four: The client develops long-term strategies for dealing with sudden 'bursts of energy' that can lead to a '*boom-bust*' effect which depletes energy once more.

Stage one: Engaging the client and understanding energy

One of the important stipulations that are recommended in helping individuals with a fatigue problem is to explain what energy is, and how it can be generated or conserved. By encouraging individuals to adopt an internal locus of control there can be self-governed symptom management, which can be liberating in certain conditions where it may be felt that they are passive receivers of care, or 'sufferers' of symptoms.

It is important to acknowledge that like pain, fatigue symptoms can dramatically hinder daily life activities or occupations (Gray and Fossey, 2003). However, since fatigue is subjective, it is hard to measure. Further, fatigue is also hard to *see* in someone else, and therefore can at times be treated rather sceptically, particularly if the fatigue is long standing (Looper and Kirmayer, 2004). This may create a desire in people to over-exert themselves in an attempt to prove that they are strong willed, and not charlatans. Once someone has been diagnosed with a fatigue causing condition such as multiple sclerosis or cancer, improvement of lifestyle factors whilst living with the condition can limit the severity of associated problems or symptoms, and divert energy into positive self-directed approaches. There are some examples of how to understand fatigue and the factors involved in Advice boxes 5.1 and 5.2.

Stage two: Identifying the personal factors influencing fatigue (Handouts 5.1 and 5.2)

It is important how energy is affected by the imbalance of occupations, and that it is not always more rest that is required. Fatigue can cause further fatigue through normal lifestyle choices. While we have all surely enjoyed a 'lazy Sunday afternoon', we rarely find ourselves invigorated at evening time following a day of rest and 'recuperation'. People commonly believe that energy is only generated by rest and sleep and yet lack activity can also cause feelings of fatigue and lethargy. So understanding the importance of a balance between quality rest and worthwhile activity is an important starting point.

Lifestyle factors such as staying up late, poor sleep, inadequate, unbalanced diet, chaotic occupational routine and stress can all play their part in making fatigue worse. Indeed, these factors are addressed comprehensively in a ten session programme for people with CFS (Cox, 2000). The programme run by occupational therapists trained in cognitive behaviour therapy, includes measuring and advising on exercise, daily activity, sleep patterns, rest and relaxation. However, Cox also goes on to advocate that throughout the lifestyle management sessions 'thoughts and feelings about their illness are explored' (p. 101). This may be appropriate in cases where fatigue is as a result of CFS; however, there is little evidence that healthy lifestyle advice needs to be supported CBT trained professionals, more, that lifestyle adjustment is likely to have positive benefits to fatigue in a variety of conditions. Comprehensive expansion on sleep, relaxation, healthy diet or work–life balance are provided in other chapters within this book.

Meaningful occupations are individual concepts (Yerxa *et al.*, 1989). For this reason, therapy may be best individualised. The use of activity/time-use charts is a commonly used approach within fatigue specialist units (DoH, 2002). One example can be photocopied (Handout 5.1) and there are instructions in Handout 5.2. This can be used to identify how individuals occupy their time, which can indicate well-being in terms of the balance of what occupations are done and why (Farnworth, 2004). However, it is revealing to have clients describe what *they* personally consider to be energy consuming and what they find is energy providing (Advice box 5.3). The life jug (Handout 5.2) identifies which occupations are draining, boring, stimulating, frustrating or stressful for that person, these can be adapted by grading as opposed to simply stopping all occupations that appear to be draining (such as driving or shopping). Essentially the combination of the life jug and activity/time-use charts allows the client to analyse their life's activities and occupations and how they are performing them, which can indicate factors that could be creating fatigue.

Establish activity and fatigue baseline

Chalder (1999) produced a fatigue scale which can be useful for measuring fatigue levels. However, it is relatively straightforward to ask the client to rate their fatigue on a scale that is relevant to them, and the best way is to rate '0' as no fatigue, and '10' being the worst they have ever felt. Comparing the activity (as recorded in the time use/activity chart) with the fatigue level identifies the factors that are creating more symptoms, then, by looking at how long, and in what way the individual did the activity, indicates how much of that activity they can tolerate before fatigue arises (Advice box 5.4). The base-line of what can be achieved without significant rises in fatigue experienced is therefore established. Having the client gradually grade and pace activities up from their baseline can help activities to be performed without exacerbating symptoms (stage 3).

Stage three: Lifestyle plan for change (grading and pacing life)

By closely examining the activity levels and the characteristics of the activities, it is possible to establish a 'lifestyle plan'. This is aimed to slowly decrease or increase the amount and manner in which the activity is performed by the client, but within a framework of a new approach towards that activity. This is known as 'grading activity'. Use Handouts 5.3 and 5.4 to describes the balance of demand and supply of energy, which can be useful when considering analysing activities of daily life. The health care professional can explore with the client the sources of energy that they have and whether these can be improved upon (see Advice box 5.5).

It may be helpful to get the client to think about how they gain quality rest in their life or to think in terms of relaxation. Understanding that physiologically the body functions differently in its relaxed state and the importance of this to energy conservation is an important step to improving energy supplies. It may be helpful to identify any strategies the client already has for relaxing and maximise these or look at learning new methods for relaxation (see Chapter 7).

Principles of grading occupations and activities (adapted from Leeds and West Yorkshire CFS Service, 2006)

Grading involves analysing activities and considering them as being made up of component parts. For example, making a meal requires muscle strength and movement, sensation, hand–eye coordination, sequencing and memory. Each component requires energy; therefore, some activities can be made easier by simply reducing the number of component parts involved. For example, preparing vegetables sitting down, is not using the additional energy required to stand. Therefore, activities can be made easier or harder depending on how they are done. We can support someone to understand that they can still do all the things they usually do, but in a different way. The client can consider returning to previously enjoyed activities that they have stopped due to fatigue.

The components of grading a task/activity are as follows: The *time* it takes to do the activity; the *distance* the body has to travel; the *speed* of doing the activity; the *strength* required to complete the task and the *complexity* of the task/activity (Advice box 5.6).

Generally most activities can be broken down in these ways, but the handout (Handout 5.4) within this chapter may be useful to back up any explanation. Even complex tasks can be broken down and reduced to the level where the client feels they can do something of that activity without feeling exhausted. For example, decorating a room could be graded in terms of

Time – giving yourself a month to complete it, or longer.
Speed – pacing the rate at which you paint the wall.
Strength – having the furniture moved by someone else beforehand.
Complexity – painting one wall at a time, using only one type and colour of paint.

Stage four: Applying 'common sense to common fatigue'

Grading of activities may increase initial experiences of fatigue, however, this should be slight as the body acclimatises to the change in how the activity is performed. Increasing activity takes on some of the principles of graded exercise programmes but with a reduced physiological impact upon the body. So there are many ways to increase activity as seen above, which do not necessarily increase heart rate for prolonged periods but can be off putting to those who already feel tired. Therefore, encourage the client to work on one occupation at a time if anxiety is expressed (see Advice box 5.7). By engaging in a graded approach, participation in meaningful daily occupations is feasible. If a significant increase in fatigue levels is experienced, it can often be pertinent to look at any underlying factors that may be making the fatigue worse (Advice box 5.8). Factors such as life stress or relationship difficulties can disturb energy levels. These areas should be seen as a problem in themselves, however, the fact that the client has responded positively to facilitating change in one area of their lives may well help them to begin to look at others.

Conclusion

Energy to engage in the meaningful occupations or tasks of life is integral to health. There are many conditions and disorders that have fatigue as one of the most troublesome symptoms. Fatigue can be addressed through lifestyle modification and change, however, severe fatigue problems require specialist interventions as lifestyle modifications alone are likely to be insufficient.

The principal strategies of lifestyle management for fatigue involve helping the client to understand that they have some control over their fatigue symptoms. Using diaries to uncover lifestyle causes for exacerbations of fatigue and analogies such as the 'jug of life' can help clients understand the drainers and energisers in their life. By grading, balancing and pacing occupations of daily life and addressing fundamental lifestyle routines and behaviours, clients should see an improvement in their symptoms.

This chapter has suggested a staged formulaic plan that can be adapted to each client; the accompanying handouts can be used to a greater or lesser extent or indeed modified to ensure client centredness. The extent of the fatigue problem may need further support in other accompanying lifestyle areas such as sleep, healthy diets and stress management. However, as with any functional problem, how the person manages and adjusts their lives can influence the degree to which someone is affected by their symptoms.

References

Barsevick, A. M., Dudley, W., Beck, S. *et al.* (2004). A randomized clinical trial of energy conservation for patients with cancer-related fatigue. *Cancer*, 100(6): 1302–1310.

Bentall, R. R., Powell, P., Nye, F. J., Edwards, R. H. (2002) Predictors of response to treatment for chronic fatigue syndrome. *British Journal of Psychiatry*, 181: 248–252.

Buchwald, D., Pearlman, T., Umali, J., Schmaling, K. and Katon, W. (1996). Functional status in patients with chronic fatigue syndrome, other fatiguing illnesses, and healthy individuals. *American Journal of Medicine*, 101(4): 364–370.

Bultmann, U., Kant, I. J. and Kasl, S. V. (2002a). Fatigue and psychological distress in the working population: psychometrics, prevalence and correlates. *Journal of Psychosomatic Research*, 52: 445–452.

Bultmann, U., Kant, I. J., Kasl, S. V. *et al.* (2002b). Lifestyle factors as risk factors for fatigue and psychological distress in the working population: prospective results from the Maastricht Cohort Study. *Journal of Occupational & Environmental Medicine*, 44(2): 116.

Carmack Taylor, C. L., de Moor, C., Basen-Engquist, K. *et al.* (2007). Moderator analyses of participants in the active for life after cancer trial: implications for physical activity group intervention studies. *Annals Behavioral Medicine*, 33(1): 99–104.

Chalder, T. (1999). *Coping with Chronic Fatigue*. London, Sheldon Press.

Chalder, T., Berelowitz, G., Pawlikowska, T. *et al.* (1993) Development of a fatigue scale. *Journal of Psychosomatic Research*, 37: 147–153.

Chalder, T., Goodman, R., Wessely, S., Hotopf, M. and Meltzer, H. (2003). Epidemiology of chronic fatigue syndrome and self-reported myalgic encephalomyelitis in 5–15 year olds: cross sectional study. *British Medical Journal*, 327: 654–655.

Clapp, L. L., Richardson, M. T., Smith, J. F. *et al.* (1999). Acute effects of thirty minutes of light-intensity, intermittent exercise on patients with chronic fatigue syndrome. *Physical Therapy*, 79: 749–756.

Clark, L. V. and White, P. D. (2005). The role of de-conditioning and therapeutic exercise in chronic fatigue syndrome (CFS). *Journal of Mental Health*, 14(3): 237–252.

Cox, D. L. (1999). Chronic fatigue syndrome – an occupational therapy programme. *Occupational Therapy International*, 6(1): 52–64.

Cox, D. L. (2000). *Occupational Therapy and Chronic Fatigue Syndrome*. London, Whurr Publishers.

Curt, G. A. (2000). The impact of fatigue on patients with cancer: overview of FATIGUE 1 and 2. *Oncologist*, 5: 9–12.

Darbishire, L., Ridsdale, L. and Seed, P. T. (2003). Distinguishing patients with chronic fatigue from those with chronic fatigue syndrome: a diagnostic study in UK primary care. *British Journal of General Practice*, 53: 441–445.

David, A., Pelosi, A., McDonald, E. *et al.* (1990). Tired, weak, or in need of rest: fatigue among general practice attenders. *British Medical Journal*, 301: 1199–1202.

De Becker, P., Roeykens, J., Reynders, M. *et al.* (2000). Exercise capacity in chronic fatigue syndrome. *Archives of Internal Medicine*, 160(21): 3270–3277.

Deale, A. and Wessely, S. (1992). Patients' perceptions of medical care in chronic fatigue syndrome. *Social Science & Medicine*, 52: 1859–1864.

DH (2002). *A Report of the CFS/ME Working Group*. London, Department of Health.

Edmonds, M., McGuire, H. and Price, J. (2004). Exercise therapy for chronic fatigue syndrome. *Cochrane Database of Systematic Reviews*, Issue 3. Chichester, John Wiley & Sons, UK DOI: 10.1002/14651858.CD003200.pub2.

Farnworth, L. (2002). Time use and disability. In Molineux, M. (ed.) *Occupation for Occupational Therapists*. London, Blackwell Publishing.

Fisk, J. D., Pontefract, A., Ritvo, P. G., Archibald, C. J. and Murray, T. J. (1994). The impact of fatigue on patients with multiple sclerosis. *Canadian Journal of Neurological Science*, 1(1): 9–14.

Fuhrer, R. and Wessely, S. (1995). The epidemiology of fatigue and depression: a French primary care study. *Psychological Medicine*, 25: 895–905.

Fukuda, K., Straus, S. E., Hickie, I. *et al.* (1994). The chronic fatigue syndrome: a comprehensive approach to its definition and study. International Chronic Fatigue Syndrome Study Group. *Annals of Internal Medicine*, 121(12): 953–959.

Fulcher, K. Y. and White, P. (2000). Strength and physicological response to exercise in patients with chronic fatigue syndrome. *Journal of Neurology Neurosurgery & Psychiatry*, 69: 302–307.

Gallagher, A. M., Thomas, J. M., Hamilton, W. T. and White, P. D. (2004). Incidence of fatigue symptoms and diagnoses presenting in UK primary care from 1990 to 2001. *Journal of the Royal Society of Medicine*, 97: 571–575.

Gallagher, A. M., Coldrick, A. R., Hedge, B., Weir, W. R. C. and White, P. D. (2005). Is the chronic fatigue syndrome an exercise phobia? A case control study. *Journal of Psychosomatic Research*, 58(4): 367–373.

Gray, M. L. and Fossey, E. M. (2003). Illness experience and occupations of people with chronic fatigue syndrome. *Australian Occupational Therapy Journal*, 50: 127.

Haines, L. C., Saidi, G. and Cooke, R. W. I. (2005). Prevalence of severe fatigue in primary care. *Archives of Disease in Childhood*, 90: 367–368.

Hann, D. M., Garovoy, N., Finkelstein, B. *et al.* (1999). Fatigue and quality of life in breast cancer patients undergoing autologous stem cell transplantation: a longitudinal comparative study. *Journal of Pain Symptom Management*, 17: 311–319.

Hickie, I. B., Hooker, A. W., Hadzi Pavlovic, D. *et al.* (1996). Fatigue in selected primary care settings: sociodemographic and psychiatric correlates. *Medical Journal Australia*, 164: 585–588.

Ingles, J. L., Eskes, G. A. and Phillips, S. J. (1999). Fatigue after stroke. *Archives of Physical Medicine and Rehabilitation*, 80(2): 173–178.

Kroenke, K., Wood, D., Mangelsdorff, D., Meier, N. and Powell, J. (1988). Chronic fatigue in primary care: prevalence, patient characteristics, and outcome. *Journal of the American Medical Association*, 260: 929–934.

Leeds and West Yorkshire CFS Service (2006). *Patient Manual on Grading Activity*. Clinical Network Coordinating Centres & Local Multidisciplinary Teams Paperless Online Documents (CFS-POD). http://www.cfspod.net/Info%20Leaflets.htm. Accessed 27 September 2007.

Loge, J. H., Abrahamsen, A. F., Ekeberg, O. and Kaasa, S. (2000). Fatigue and psychiatric morbidity among Hodgkin's disease survivors. *Journal of Pain Symptom Management*, 19: 91–99.

Looper, K. J. and Kirmayer, L. J. (2004). Perceived stigma in functional somatic syndromes and comparable medical conditions. *Journal of Psychosomatic Research*, 57(4): 373–378.

Mathiowetz, V., Matuska, K. M. and Murphy, M. E. (2001). Efficacy of an energy conservation course for persons with multiple sclerosis. *Archives of Physical Medicine and Rehabilitation*, 82: 449–456.

McCrone, P., Darbishire, N. L., Ridsdale, L. and Seed, P. (2003) The economic cost of chronic fatigue and chronic fatigue syndrome in UK primary care. *Psychological Medicine*, 33: 253–261.

McDermott, C., Richards, S. C. M., Ankers, S. *et al.* (2004). An evaluation of a chronic fatigue lifestyle management programme focusing on the outcome of return to work or training. *British Journal of Occupational Therapy*, 67 (6): 269–273.

McNeely, M. L., Campbell, K. L., Rowe, B. H. *et al.* (2006). Effects of exercise on breast cancer patients and survivors: a systematic review and meta-analysis. *Canadian Medical Association Journal*, 175: 34–41.

Moss-Morris, Rona, Sharon, Cynthia, Tobin, Roseanne, Baldi, James, C. 2005. A randomized controlled graded exercise trial for chronic fatigue syndrome: outcomes and mechanisms of change. *Journal of Health Psychology*, 10: 245–259.

NICE (National Institute for Health and Clinical Excellence) (2007). *Chronic Fatigue Syndrome/Myalgic Encephalomyelitis (or Encephalopathy): Diagnosis and Management of CFS/ME in Adults and Children.* London, NICE, http://guidance.nice.org.uk/CG053

Nijs, J., Vanherberghen, K., Duquet, W. and De Meirleir, K. (2004). Chronic fatigue syndrome: lack of association between pain-related fear of movement and exercise capacity and disability. *Physical Therapy*, 84: 696–705.

Pawlikowska, T., Chalder, T., Hirsch, S. R. *et al.* (1994). Population-based study of fatigue and psychological distress. *British Medical Journal*, 308: 763–766.

Portenoy, R. K. and Itri, L. M. (1999). Cancer-related fatigue: guidelines for evaluation and management. *Oncologist*, 4: 1–10.

Price, R. K., North, C. S., Wessely, S. and Fraser, V.J. (1992). Estimating the prevalence of chronic fatigue syndrome and associated symptoms in the community. *Public Health Reports*, 107: 514–522.

Puetz, T., Beasman, K. M., O'Connor, P. J. (2006). The effect of cardiac rehabilitation exercise programs on feelings of energy and fatigue: a meta-analysis of research from 1945 to 2005. *European Journal of Cardiovascular Prevention & Rehabilitation*, 13(6): 886–893.

Ranjith, G. (2005). Epidemiology of chronic fatigue syndrome. *Occupational Medicine*, 55: 13–19.

Resnick, H. E., Carter, E. A., Aloia, M. and Phillips, B. (2006). Cross-sectional relationship of reported fatigue to obesity, diet, and physical activity: results from the Third National Health and Nutrition Examination Survey. *Journal of Clinical Sleep Medicine*, 15(2): 163–9.

Ridsdale, L., Godfrey, E., Chalder, T. *et al.* (2001). Chronic fatigue in general practice: is counselling as good as cognitive behaviour therapy? A UK randomised trial. *British Journal of General Practice*, 51(462): 19–24.

Roessler, Christa, Barling, Jenny Dephoff, Megan, Johnson, and Terri, Sweeney, S. (2004). Developing and implementing lifestyle management programs with people with multiple sclerosis. *Occupational Therapy in Health care*, 17(3–4): 97–114.

Samaha, E., Lal, S., Samaha, N. and Wyndham, J. (2007). Psychological, lifestyle and coping contributors to chronic fatigue in shift-worker nurses. *Journal of Advanced Nursing*, 59(3): 221–232.

Schwartz, A. L., Nail, L. M., Chen, S. *et al.* (2000). Fatigue patterns observed in patients receiving chemotherapy and radiotherapy. *Cancer Investigation*, 18(1): 11–19.

Sharpe, M. (1998). Cognitive behavior therapy for chronic fatigue syndrome: efficacy and implications. *American Journal of Medicine*, 105: S104–S109.

Sharpe, M. (2006). The symptom of generalised fatigue. *Practical Neurology*, 6: 72–77.

Skapinakis, P., Lewis, G. and Meltzer, H. (2003). Clarifying the relationship between explained chronic fatigue and psychiatric morbidity: results from a community survey in Great Britain. *International Review of Psychiatry*, 15: 57–64.

Smith, S. and Sullivan, K. (2003). Examining the influence of biological and psychological factors on cognitive performance in chronic fatigue syndrome; a randomized, double-blind, placebo-controlled, crossover study. *International Journal of Behavior Medicine*, 10: 162–173.

Smith, Robert C., Lein, Catherine, Collins, Clare *et al.* (2003). Treating patients with medically unexplained symptoms in primary care. *Journal of General Internal Medicine*, June, 18(6): 478–489.

Stamm, T., Wright, J., Machold, K. P., Sadlo, G. and Smolen, J. (2004). Occupational balance of women with rheumatoid arthritis: a qualitative study. *Musculoskeletal Care*, 2(2): 101–112.

Steultjens, E. M. J., Dekker, J., Bouter, L. M. *et al.* (2004). *Occupational Therapy for Multiple Sclerosis (Cochrane Review)*. In: The Cochrane Library, Issue 1. Chichester, UK, John Wiley & Sons.

Surakka, J., Romberg, A., Ruutiainen, J. *et al.* (2004). Effects of aerobic and strength exercise on motor fatigue in men and women with multiple sclerosis: a randomized controlled trial. *Clinical Rehabilitation*, 18: 737–746.

Troy, N. W. (1999). A comparison of fatigue and energy levels at 6 weeks and 14 to 19 months postpartum. *Clinical Nursing Research*, 8: 135–152.

Turnbull, N., Shaw, E. J., Baker, R. *et al.* (2007). *Diagnosis and Management of Chronic Fatigue Syndrome/Myalgic Encephalomyelitis (or Encephalopathy) in Adults and Children*. London, Royal College of General Practitioners.

Van Houdenhovea, B., Neerinckxb, E., Onghenac, P., Lysensa, R. and Vertommenc, H. (2001). Premorbid 'overactive' lifestyle in chronic fatigue syndrome and fibromyalgia. An etiological factor or proof of good citizenship? *Journal of Psychosomatic Research*, 51: 571–576.

Von Korff, M. and Tiemens, B. (2000). Individualized stepped care of chronic illness. *Western Journal of Medicine*, 172(2): 133–137.

Ward, N. and Winters, S. (2003). Results of a fatigue management programme in multiple sclerosis. *British Journal of Nursing*, 12(18): 1075–1080.

Ward, S. E. (1993). The common sense model: an organizing framework for knowledge development in nursing. *Scholarly Inquiry for Nursing Practice*, 7: 79–90.

Wearden, A. J. and Chew-Graham, C. (2006). Managing chronic fatigue syndrome in UK primary care: challenges and opportunities. *Chronic Illness*, 2(2): 143–153.

Wessely, S., Chalder, T., Hirsch, S., Wallace, P. and Wright, D. (1997). The prevalence and morbidity of chronic fatigue and chronic fatigue syndrome: a prospective primary care study. *American Journal of Public Health*, 87(9): 1449–1455.

Wessely, S., Hotopf, M. and Sharpe, M. (1998). *Chronic Fatigue and Its Syndromes*. Oxford, Oxford University Press.

Whiting, P., Bagnall, A. M., Sowden, A. J. *et al.* (2001). Interventions for the treatment and management of chronic fatigue syndrome: a systematic review. *Journal of American Medical Association*, 286(11): 1360–1368.

Woodward, R., Broom, D. and Legge, D. (1995). Diagnosis in chronic illness: disabling or enabling – the case of chronic fatigue syndrome. *Journal of the Royal Society Medicine*, 88: 325–329.

Yerxa, E., Clark, F., Jackson, J., Parham, D., Pierce, D., Stein, C. and Zemke, R. (1989) An introduction to occupational Science, a foundation for occupational therapy in the twenty first century. *Occupational Therapy in Health Care*, 6(4): 1–17.

All of the following handouts and advice boxes can be found as individual pdfs on the website at www.blackwellpublishing.com/thew

Advice box 5.1 The psychology of energy

It is usual and common for fatigue levels to fluctuate, this is the normal pattern in healthy individuals. When people experience an increase in their fatigue they may wait for a day for their energy to return, so they cancel or avoid trips/visits/holidays in an attempt to improve subjective fatigue. However, this approach denies pleasurable experiences, which can be energising.

The psychology of energy is such that we tend to always have more energy for the things we want/desire to do. Helping clients to understand this relationship is important particularly when exploring factors that can make fatigue worse.

Advice box 5.2 Analogies to help understand energy

Analogies can help people engage in managing their energy. The following simple analogy is useful to illustrate how energy can be used up.

> Imagine two men at traffic lights, in identical makes of car. One man is revving his engine at the lights, has clearly not looked after the car, as it is blowing out smoke. The lights turn to green, the cars set off, the non-serviced car is soon out of sight. After 5 minutes, the more slow and well-maintained car pulls along side the other, which unfortunately has crashed and burned. He offers a lift to the unfortunate now, car-less man, he turns down the offer, as he is never going to step in that type of car again.

Ask the client if this sounds familiar to how they tend to behave, highlight the similarities of the car being like the body, you need to treat your body like a precious commodity; if you do not, it breaks down, if you burn up energy rapidly, you run low on fuel more quickly, and lastly, it is not the body, but how you use it! This is useful if someone attributes their condition to their age or circumstances.

Advice box 5.3 Using analogies: The jug of life and energy (see Handout 5.2)

The analogy is one of energy being seen as water in a jug (which represents the body). Draw a jug on a sheet of A4 size paper (or use the handout version). Describe the jug as representing the body. The water that is in it is energy. Ask the client to put a line on where they see the water level in the jug in terms of energy level in their life.

If there is a pre-existing condition (such as cancer/multiple sclerosis, etc.) this could be depicted as a crack in the side of the jug, which essentially is a constant drain or leak of energy, which has to be compensated for. This helps people to see that although they have a medical condition, the problem in terms of fatigue can be addressed.

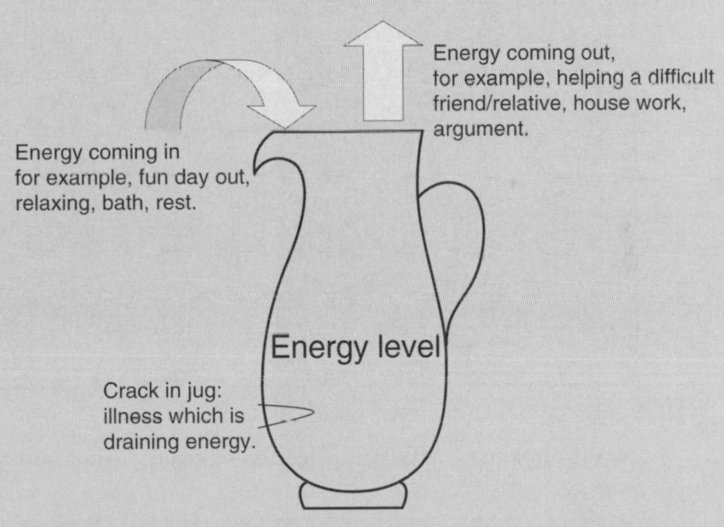

NB: Can have several arrows, the arrows are sized in accordance with how energy consuming or energy providing the element is.

Advice box 5.3 Continued

The next step is to ask the client to draw what they see as being the energy consuming elements of their life. This is represented by an arrow going from inside to outside the jug, literally showing where the individual is pouring their energy. This could be work, children, household chores, and can be as much detailed as the client sees fit. The extent of how energy consuming the element is represented by an arrow being either broad or narrow.

When the drawing is complete, explore the important issues. If the client feels they need to keep the energy consuming elements in their lives, look at grading and adapting them (stages 2 and 3). If the client chooses to keep their lifestyle as it currently stands, ask them to look at increasing the pleasurable/energising elements.

Advice box 5.4 Understanding energy diaries

Ask the client to complete the diary to establish a 'baseline value'. This baseline is the amount or extent that an activity is performed before fatigue occurs, for example, if on the client's chart it is evident that driving for 1 hour has resulted in pain and fatigue, but half an hour appears not to increase fatigue, then there will be a baseline somewhere in between. This may mean, for example, reducing the time spent driving without a break. Ask the client to identify any routines, and if there is a 'little and often' approach to daily life. Indicate if there is any evidence of 'boom and bust' where the client is overdoing it one day and then undergoing things in reaction to increased fatigue the next day. Consistency and routine is important here. Establishing baseline routines, for example, set bed times, wake times, reducing naps during the day, (see Chapter 6) or by integrating sensible eating times, as well as getting other occupations into a healthy balanced routine can help to prevent 'boom–crash' behaviour.

The charts may pick up on emotional issues, such as arguments, or stressful events. The client may choose to explore these, or wait until they 'feel better' to explore these at a later date.

Advice box 5.5 Analyzing results of energy diary and jug of life and energy

Ask the patient to make a list of the main demands upon their energy and the main sources of energy that they have. The client may identify possibilities for change, such as reducing the levels of demand or increasing opportunities for pleasure/relaxation. These areas can then be developed into specific goals as part of the lifestyle plan.

Advice box 5.6 How to grade activities to limit energy use

How to modify the activity to gain energy in terms of

1. Time. The longer the period of time spent on an activity the more energy it will require. Time is the easiest measure to apply. Through setting time limits for each activity, the individual can identify their baseline and gradually increase the time periods allocated to each task. The person needs to be able to tolerate the activity for the time agreed without experiencing subsequent increased fatigue. In other words, when driving long distances, you may have to incorporate rest breaks so that you are not at the wheel for too long.

2. Distance. Distance is a more appropriate measure for any activity which involves motion, such as walking, swimming, driving, and so on. Markers can be used to indicate the distance to be used as a baseline, for example, walking to a specific landmark or swimming a number of lengths of the pool. People can often be focused on reaching the end point, such as getting to the local shop, and may not accept the need to work gradually towards this, such as only walking part way along the street, resting and returning.

3. Speed. Speed is the combination of time and distance, the ability to perform the task faster. It is often the case with fatigue that 'more haste makes less speed'. By pacing and pegging back speed, fewer mistakes are made, and the available energy stretches further. This is a lot like revving the engine of a car; you need to drive conservatively when you want to keep more petrol in the tank.

4. Strength. This relates to muscle power and stamina. Muscle bulk decreases through inactivity. People who have previously maintained high levels of physical activity may be frustrated by the effects of muscle de-conditioning. Strength can only be regained in response to the demands of an activity, through gradually increasing the muscle power needed for the task. For example, strength in the upper limbs can be increased through the amount of weight carried in shopping bags.

5. Complexity. Complexity concerns the number of factors influencing the activity, for instance, how many senses are involved, and are they all involved at the same time? For example, driving is a complex task, whereas something like watching television is not. One involves concentrating and using all the senses and physical components of the body at the same time. By making the task less complex, the task may be more achievable and less fatiguing (e.g. driving in less traffic or using an automatic car).

Advice box 5.7 Using the activity diary with the grading advice

By examining the activity diary, ask the client to choose one activity that they are wanting to do more of, but are presently unable to do due to lack of energy. Ask them to examine first how could they complete the task by allowing more time for it, over less distance, incorporating a rest, what could make the task/activity less onerous in terms of strength required, how could the activity be simplified and how could they slow down the speed at which they do it.

Advice box 5.8 Advising after relapse

If improvement has been achieved, and there has been an increase in activities, without an increase in symptoms, the temptation may be to consider that the fatigue problem is 'cured'. The client may need support to see that it is their self-management that has created the improvement, and a return to the 'old habits' may see a return to problem fatigue.

If there is a relapse in symptoms, ask for another chart to be completed, and look for any 'overdoing' of activities well over the 'baseline' and look for 'extreme' days, where one day is full of rest and sedentary activity and the next, in comparison, is the opposite. This can lead to a poorly controlled life once again. Ask the client to keep to the 'little and often' rule for all activities for a while, and then gently increase the amount of activity once again. Alternatively, complete the life jug to ascertain if a recent life change is acting as an energy drainer.

Handout 5.1 Individual energy and life diary

Hours of day	Monday	Tuesday	Wednesday	Thursday	Friday	Saturday	Sunday
7–8 a.m.							
8–9 a.m.							
9–10 a.m.							
10–11 a.m.							
11 a.m.–12 p.m.							
12–1 p.m.							
1–2 p.m.							
2–3 p.m.							
3–4 p.m.							
4–5 p.m.							
5–6 p.m.							
6–7 p.m.							
7–8 p.m.							
8–9 p.m.							
9–10 p.m.							
10–11 p.m.							

If you engage in activities of occupations later than 11 p.m., please comment here: also, comment on quality of sleep (if poor) following the day's activities. Record your fatigue levels on the hour, on a scale of 0 = no fatigue to 10 = worse fatigue ever experienced.

Handout 5.2 Understanding fatigue and energy

Fatigue can be disabling, and very frustrating to manage, as it is difficult to measure, or for others to *see.* Some fatigue is normal, and is to be expected (such as that following a late night). As it is so common, most people have learnt their own ways and means of dealing with it. Including going to bed early, having an afternoon nap, playing sport. However, you have been given this handout to help you manage fatigue that is *abnormal* for you, that you are not able to manage in your usual way.

Making your energy work for you. First, you need to identify the factors that appear to be making your fatigue worse; these are usually related to how you manage the energy that you have available. Completing the time-use diary can help (Handout 5.1). In terms of using the energy diary, you will need to keep an accurate, continuous record of *what you do in each hour* for at least a week. The week that you complete this should be a 'typical week' (not whilst you are away on holiday, for example). This is in order to pick up on patterns of lifestyle that may be hindering your ability to create or conserve energy.

You may see some patterns emerging, which you know are not going to be helpful such as an erratic sleep pattern or lack of meal times. You may have to combine several life changes for at least 2 weeks before you notice a difference.

The jug of life and energy. The following analogy helps you to identify where your energy is coming from, and where and how you are spending the majority of your energy, it also indicates whether something in your life is causing you more fatigue than it should do.

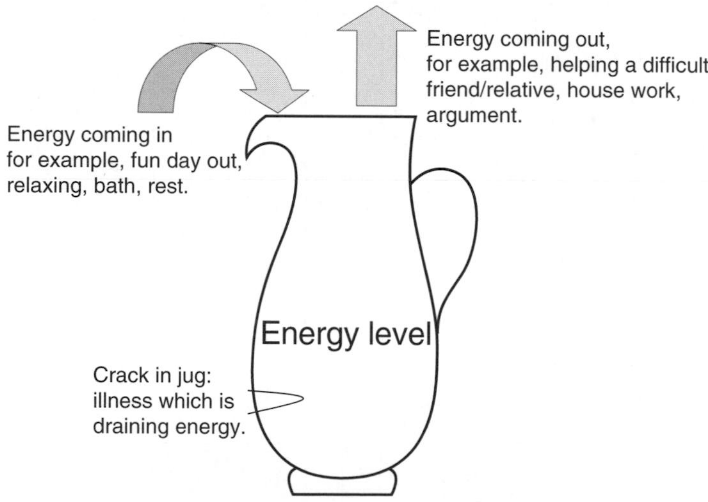

NB: Can have several arrows, the arrows are sized in accordance with how energy consuming or energy providing the element is.

Imagine your energy is like water, and the jug is your body/mind/soul containing the energy. Indicate on the jug (draw a line) where your current average energy is in terms of water in the jug. If you have a diagnosed condition which is one cause of the fatigue, represent this with a crack in the jug, if you feel this crack is the only cause of fatigue, make the crack in the jug more substantial, if the crack is only one potential cause, make it less large, and so on.

Energy coming into the jug is represented by arrows coming in and energy going out of the jug is represented by arrows going out. Draw the size of the arrow commensurate with the amount of energy coming in and out.

Remember, that energy is not only a physical thing! There are a great many things in our lives that can cause energy depletion; anxiety uses adrenaline, which in turn burns up energy. Worry leads to anxiety symptoms, so having a few hours of worry can feel like you have run a marathon.

Some of the things that can be a source of energy: 'energy drainers'	**Some of the things that can give you energy: 'energy suppliers'**
Looking after someone who is ill	Taking time out to do 'own interests/hobbies'
Driving long distances	Rest during the day
Child care	Sleeping adequately during the night
Housework	Having fun
Work/employment	Socialising
Travel	A good friend to talk to
Living with someone you do not *get al*ong with	Supportive partner/family member
Evening study	Work/employment that you enjoy

No two people are alike, therefore these lists are merely examples, but often people report that the most energy consuming elements of their lives are the emotional ones. By drawing in the arrows at the top of the jug to represent the energy coming in and out, it may be possible to see if there are more drains on your energy than supply.

This means that you have a choice, either to modify or adapt the way that you are managing the issues, activities, and so on, that are acting as drains, or increase the amount of energy suppliers in your life. For example, you are spending a lot of your energy supporting others (friends and family) but getting no social or 'fun' time for yourself.

Handout 5.2 Continued

The jug will start to empty, it needs to be replenished; otherwise, at some point you will run out of energy altogether so that you will be unable to supply energy to others or to the activities you have described.

This kind of 'run dry' is when you get so exhausted that you become medically unwell, and you may trigger off a variety of conditions, or certainly exacerbate underlying ones.

When you have little energy in your jug, to start with, the way forward, would be to explore how to manage the small amount of energy that you have, and try to adapt the way in which you do things, and ensure you are open to activities that could give you pleasure and therefore fill your jug with energy.

Handout 5.3 Supply and demand

A useful way to understand the importance of balancing out and grading activity is to use the concept of measuring scales. On one side of the scales is the energy supply and measured against this on the other side is all the demands on that energy.

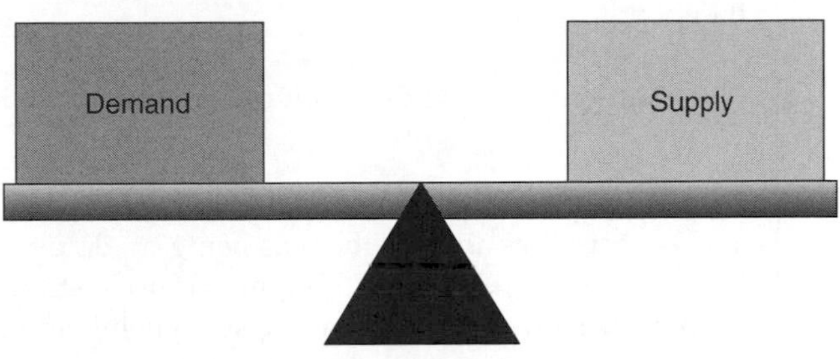

Supply. There are many aspects of life that contribute to our energy supplies, such as nutrition, sleep and pleasure. Consider what are the current energy providers that supply you with energy, can these be improved upon? For example, if seeing your friends for a coffee gives you pleasure and is a source of relaxation, then perhaps you should do more of this. Resting is not always the best source of energy supply; even sitting watching TV, although sedentary, involves emotions and the effort of concentration. Over-resting can lead to more fatigue, so it may be easier to look for opportunities for mini-breaks or pauses during or between tasks, as these give the opportunity for the body to slow its rhythm whilst not over-resting.

Demand. The demands on energy can be positive and negative and come from lots of different sources, such as family, work, running a house, and so on. They can also come from the pressure of trying to meet expectations or standards. It can therefore be helpful to identify whether any of these things could be done differently, could anyone help with these demands, or do they need to be done at all! Sometimes, we have demands that we can do nothing to change. If it really is the case that they cannot be managed differently, then you might need to consider how to increase the supply to counteract the demand, such as the financial situation or support from others.

Handout 5.4 It is not the what, but the how

Consider this: which activity would you say exhausts you the most?

Would you say that driving is the most exhausting? Or playing tennis? Or reading a complicated book? Well, you have probably guessed it.

It depends

It depends on *how* you do it, not really the activity itself.

Grading and pacing life's activities and occupations. Grading is where you analyse activities and see them as being made up of component parts. For example, making a meal requires muscle strength and movement, sensation, hand–eye coordination, sequencing and memory. Each component requires energy; therefore, some activities can be made easier by simply reducing the number of component parts involved. For example, if you prepare the vegetables sitting down, you are not using the additional energy required to stand. Therefore, activities can be made easier or harder depending on how they are done. By understanding that you can still do all the things you usually do, but in a different way, hopefully you can get back to what you like and want to do.

The best way to break things down is by looking at your activities in the following ways:

1. *Time*

How long does it take you to do an activity?
Can you do this time regularly or are you pushing yourself to do this on a better day?
The longer the period of time spent on an activity, the more energy it will require. Time is the easiest measure to apply. Through setting time limits for each activity, you can identify what you can manage without fatigue and gradually increase the time periods allocated to each task. You need to be able to tolerate the activity for the time agreed without experiencing subsequent increased fatigue. In other words, when driving long distances, you may have to incorporate rest breaks so that you are not at the wheel for too long.

2. *Distance*

How far can you go?
Distance is a more appropriate measure for any activity which involves motion, such as walking, swimming, driving, and so on. Markers can be used to indicate the distance to be used as a baseline, for example walking to a specific landmark or swimming a number

of lengths of the pool. This can gradually be made a more distant marker, as your tolerance increases. However, by incorporating rests, it may be possible to reach the point you want to, but it will include incorporating a different method to get there.

3. *Speed*

How fast are you doing the activity?
Speed is the combination of time and distance, the ability to perform the task faster. It is often the case with fatigue that 'more haste makes less speed'. By pacing and pegging back speed, less mistakes are made, and the available energy stretches further. This is a lot like revving the engine of a car; you need to drive conservatively when you want to keep more petrol in the tank.

4. *Strength*

How much power do you need to do this task?
This relates to muscle power and stamina. Muscle bulk decreases through inactivity. People who have previously maintained high levels of physical activity may be frustrated by the effects of muscle de-conditioning. Strength can only be regained in response to the demands of an activity, through gradually increasing the muscle power needed for the task. For example, strength in the upper limbs can be increased through the amount of weight carried in shopping bags.

5. *Complexity*

Is this a simple activity or are there lots of different things that you need to do the same time?

How many senses are involved, and are they all involved at the same time? For example, driving is a complex task, whereas reading a simple magazine article is not. One involves concentrating and using senses and physical components of the body all at the same time. By making the task less complex, the task may be more achievable and less fatiguing (e.g. driving in less traffic or in automatic car, etc).

Generally, most activities in your life can be adapted: if you want to keep them in your life, it is down to you and how you choose to do it.

6. *Good Sleep – The Life Enhancer*

Miranda Thew

Introduction

We spend around a third of our lives asleep. A satisfying nights sleep can be seen to enhance daily occupational performance and contribute to a sense of well being. Yet sleep disturbance is common in the adult population, and it is usually accompanied by behavioural/psychological and cognitive effects (Wlodarczyk *et al.*, 2002; Scott *et al.*, 2006). Insomnia is the most common disturbance, and is associated with detriments in physical and mental health (Akerstedt and Nilsson, 2003; Groeger *et al.*, 2004; Morgenthaler *et al.*, 2006). Insomnia is defined as a problem with falling or staying asleep, or where the quality of sleep is not refreshing and restorative (American Academy of Sleep Medicine, 2005). Most insomniacs can be effectively assessed and treated within an office setting. A multidimensional approach to treatment is recommended, including a range of pragmatic sleep hygiene measures, and cognitive behavioural therapy (CBT) techniques (Vgontzas and Kales, 1999; Summers *et al.*, 2006). The current evidence suggests that there is a relative advantage of psychotherapies (such as CBT) over pharmacological therapy in that sleep not only improves, but the effects are longer lasting (Morin, 2006).

Most adults experience periods of poor sleep compared to their normal pattern, however most do not consult health care practitioners, relying instead on herbal remedies and self-help strategies such as relaxation (Morin *et al.*, 2006; Neubauer, 2006). Difficulty with sleeping is not only a primary disorder in its own right, but it is also commonly one of the most troublesome symptoms in a wide range of disorders and illnesses (Davidson *et al.*, 2002; Suka *et al.*, 2003). Yet sleep practices can be modified to good effect even in cases where there is a common cause of sleep deprivation, such as with early post-partum women (Stremler *et al.*, 2006).

A plethora of resources are available to professional and general public alike, which, although useful, can be overwhelming. Some web-based resources appear to base their products and advice on rather limited evidence. Any resources recommended in this chapter, most closely correspond to peer-reviewed evidence and are those that not commercially biased.

Literature concerned with non-pharmacological treatment for insomnia frequently refers to 'sleep hygiene rules' or regimen, which despite being over 30 years old, outlines practical advice for problems in sleeping (Hauri, 1977) and is still applicable today. Indeed, these rules are applied in a range of treatment trials, including those for underlying conditions such as diabetes and hypertension (Chasens, 2007; Morin *et al.*, 2007). These practical self-help tips are referred to in this chapter, however, despite their popularity, remain unsubstantiated in terms of single efficacy for primary or secondary insomnias (Morgenthaler *et al.*, 2006). For sleep disorders requiring specialist medical intervention, the advice in this chapter can be considered complementary.

This chapter aims to identify the kinds of routines that are helpful or unhelpful to sleep, as well as pointing out approaches to changing lifestyle behaviours that could be perpetuating any sleep inhibitory habits. The handouts include a sleep diary to elucidate the extent of the sleep problem and help (with printed factual information) challenge any exaggerated or problematic beliefs and thoughts regarding sleep duration and quality. For this reason, and whether or not insomnia is of primary origin or of organic nature, or as a result of lifestyle, this chapter equips the health and social care professional with a fundamental understanding of the characteristics, causes and strategies that are influential in getting a 'good night's sleep'.

Sleep and health

Poor quality and quantity of sleep are associated with reduced daily occupational function and quality of life (Zammit *et al.*, 1999; Sateia *et al.*, 2000; Akerstedt and Nilsson, 2003). Even relatively small reductions in sleep quality can affect health and performance (Akerstedt and Nilsson, 2003). Sleep problems in the US result in $16 billion in annual health care expenses and $50 billion in lost productivity (Carmona, 2004). Where sleep is considered to be of good quality and lasting an average of 7 hours, there is an association with increased satisfaction with life and decreased tension, depression, anger, fatigue and confusion (Pilcher *et al.*, 1997). Kronholm and colleagues (2006) suggest that sleep and lifestyle are synonymous:

> Sleep duration can be considered as a lifestyle factor that is modulated and influenced by a range of background factors or a factor determined by the underlying health condition and genotype of an individual. (p. 277)

The large-scale study by Akerstedt and colleagues (2002) found that old age, being female, having high body mass index (BMI) and a lack of exercise can all contribute to insomnia. Other studies have correlated a significant association between short sleep duration and being overweight (Seicean *et al.*, 2007). Chronic sleep problems are common in diabetes sufferers (Spiegel *et al.*, 2005). Sleep disordered breathing (sleep apnoea) is associated with diabetes even when other risk factors (such as being overweight) are accounted for (Reichmuth *et al.*, 2005). Specific sleep disorders are associated with increasing the risk of fatal conditions, for example, heart attack (Marin *et al.*, 2005).

Sleep deprivation effects on health

In mammals, sleep repairs neuronal damage and/or reorganisation of metabolic processes in the brain, conversely, the rest of the body apart from rest, gains little (Savage and West, 2007). However, where sleep deprivation is measured, it leads to increased levels of generalised fatigue which can interfere with performance in daily life particularly cognitive functioning (Van Dongen *et al.*, 2003). One study found that if sleep is reduced by as little as 1.3–1.5 hours in one night's worth of sleep, the resultant reduction in daytime alertness can be as much as 32% (Bonnet and Arand, 1995). Hypertension is associated with poor sleep; with one study of a large sample of adults in the US suggesting that subjects who reported averaging 5 or less hours of sleep per night, were at an increased risk for developing the condition (Gangwisch *et al.*, 2006). Suka *et al.* (2003) also found there was a correlation between sleep deprivation and hypertension. It could be argued, therefore, that resolving the effects of sleep deprivation not only increases quality of life but is a lifestyle factor that is as relevant as other treatments or prevention programmes (e.g. antihypertensives, dietary advice or exercise) for hypertension.

A large-scale recent study found that chronic insomnia has been found to be a factor in the incidence of anxiety disorders although less likely for depression (Neckelmann *et al.*, 2007). The findings of Neckelmann and colleagues indicate that successful treatment of chronic insomnia may therefore help prevent an anxiety disorder from developing. Akerstedt *et al.* (2002) found that the inability to stop worrying about work during free time may be an important link in the relation between stress and sleep. This can suggest that there is an element of a cyclical problem, where the stress of every day life can interfere with sleep, and that poor quality of sleep can cause detrimental effects on the ability to cope with every day life events.

The characteristics of sleep

In understanding the pattern and characteristics of sleep, the health care professional can not only assess the extent of the problem but also advise wherein that problem may lie. For example, brief night-time waking is common, but attention being paid to what is considered a harmless and frequent occurrence, can lead to anxiety about waking and therefore prolong the period of being awake (Summers *et al.*, 2006). By taking an educational and factual approach in advising clients, the health professional can help challenge any irrational beliefs about the amount, and the way in which sleep is being taken.

What is sleep?

Many books and web resources describe the pattern and stages of sleep, and it becomes therefore redundant to be too detailed here, more that a brief explanation of the typical characteristics of sleep can set the scene to people prior to completing sleep diaries. Many species sleep, and it is an instinctive reversible behaviour (Carskdon and Dement, 2000) which is generally required to perform a wide range of tasks whether consolidated from past learning or recently learned (Greene and Siegel, 2004). Generally, most adults sleep for an average of 6.7 hours for White women to 5.1 hours for Black men (Lauderdale *et al.*, 2006). Although mean time in bed can be longer (7.5 hours), mean sleep duration is 6.1 hours. Typically women sleep more than men, and quality and quantity of sleep decreases with age (Walsleben *et al.*, 2004). Socioeconomic status is only weakly associated with time spent in bed, although

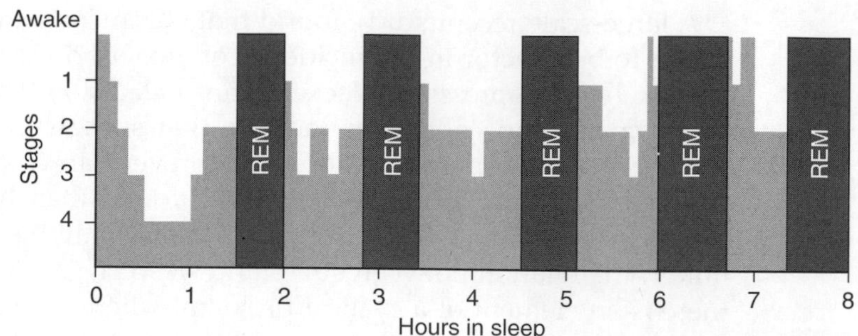

Fig. 6.1 States and stages of sleep (Source: *Let Sleep Work for You,* National Sleep Foundation, 2007. www.sleepfoundation.org).

those on higher incomes/education tend to spend less time in bed and sleep fewer hours (Lauderdale *et al.*, 2006). Usually, quality of sleep is influenced by the pattern of recent sleep (e.g. a previous late night), circadian rhythm (body clock), external factors such as room temperature, and intrinsic factors such as alcohol consumption or clinical symptoms, for example, pain (Summers *et al.*, 2006; Murphy and Delanty, 2007).

Sleep stages

There are two types of sleep: rapid eye movement (REM) sleep and non-rapid eye movement (NREM) sleep. With four basic stages a cyclical pattern exists (see Figure 6.1), where each cycle lasts approximately 90–110 minutes. There are several episodes when sleep is so light that it is often likely that individuals can awaken. The earlier sleep cycles contain more deep NREM sleep, with the REM and stage 1–2 NREM sleep occurring later (usually in the morning). Each stage lowers the individual into deeper form of sleep, with only a subtle difference between relaxation and stage 1 sleep.

Stage 1 (NREM)

Stage 1 is similar to that of deep relaxation, with muscle tone easing, however, usually the individual is more or less conscious but awakens easily, particularly in response to external stimuli. Possibly this stage offers little advantage to the body other than rest alone. Often people deny that they have actually fallen asleep. This stage usually is quite brief (10 minutes or so). Sleep advice often appertains to helping the body to move from this stage of sleep into deeper sleep stages (Rechtschaffen and Siegel, 1999).

Stage 2 (NREM)

In stage 2, the body falls into a deeper state of relaxation, this is known as 'delta sleep' due to the corresponding brain waves. It is characterised by the body having muscle tone mixed with periods of muscle relaxation and decreases in blood pressure, metabolism, cardiac activity and body temperature. In stage 2, the body is preparing for deep sleep, by becoming more detached from the outside world, even though external noise can still cause wakening.

Stage 3 and stage 4 (NREM)

These stages are a much deeper form of sleep than stages 1 and 2, occurring 30 minutes after falling asleep. Characteristically, people can sleep walk and talk, and if a person is woken up, they will be quite disorientated and possibly need some minutes to regain normal function. In this stage the body is most at rest, and bodily activity most reduced.

REM sleep

This type of sleep stands out from the other stages of sleep, in that although muscles are effectively 'paralysed' (hence, why sleep walking does not occur), heart rate increases, with a resultant rise in blood pressure. Breathing becomes rapid and shallow, and the brain is as active as when awake with eyes darting back and forth (lending the name of 'REM' to this stage). REM sleep causes dreaming, and if woken, the individual can recall their dream, whereas, if woken from NREM sleep, there is no recall. Infants spend longer in REM sleep than adults, which can explain why children often complain of 'night terrors'.

For a more comprehensive guide on sleep characteristics particularly for client use, refer to the following websites:

Royal College of Psychiatrists: www.rcpsych.ac.uk/pdf/sleep.pdf
Psychology World: http://web.umr.edu/~psyworld/sleep_stages.htm
National Sleep Foundation: http://www.sleepfoundation.org.

Sleep disorders

There are a large number of sleep disorders, but the most common and well known are those listed in Table 6.1 (International Classification of Diseases – ICD-10). Although a more expansive categorisation (International Classification of Sleeping Disorders – ICSD) is obtainable online http://www.absm.org/PDF/ICSD.pdf (American Academy of Sleep Medicine, 2005). This 600 page document itemises and classifies 90 disorders of sleep, including those that are pathological, such as Narcolepsy or Obstructive Sleep Apnoea Syndrome (see Box 6.1). Many of these problems may require specialist intervention, and referral via a general practitioner (GP) is advisable.

Insomnia

Insomnia can be characterised by being a habitual, nightly occurrence of unsatisfactory quantity and quality of sleep, and being judged to be mild to severe (American Academy of Sleep Medicine, 2005).

Table 6.1 ICD-10 codes for sleep disorders.

ICD-10 code	International classification of diseases
F51	Non-organic sleep disorders
F51.0	Non-organic insomnia
F51.1	Non-organic hypersomnia
F51.2	Non-organic disorder of the sleep–wake schedule
F51.3	Sleep walking (somnambulism)
F51.4	Sleep terrors (night terrors)
F51.5	Nightmares
F51.8	Other non-organic sleep disorder
F51.9	Non-organic sleep disorder, unspecified
G47	Sleep disorders
G47.0	Disorders of initiating and maintaining sleep (insomnias)
G47.1	Disorders of excessive somnolence (hypersomnias)
G47.2	Disorders of the sleep–wake schedule
G47.3	Sleep apnoea
G47.4	Narcolepsy and cataplexy
G47.8	Other sleep disorder
G47.9	Sleep disorder, unspecified

Note: Data according to International Statistical Classification of Diseases and Related Health Problems, 10th Revision, Version for 2007, World Health Organization.

Box 6.1 Essential features of common organic sleep disorders

Narcolepsy

> ... is a disorder of unknown etiology that is characterized by excessive sleepiness that typically is associated with cataplexy and other REM sleep phenomena, such as sleep paralysis and hypnagogic hallucinations.
>
> (American Academy of Sleep Medicine, 2005, p. 38)

Narcolepsy most commonly occurs in the teenage or early adult years, with the severity of disorder lessening with age. The sleepiness tends to manifest itself in frequent episodes of brief naps during the day, with consequential deleterious effects on occupational performance. Cataplexy describes a sudden loss of skeletal muscle tone, without loss of consciousness, thus rendering the sufferer unable to function. In a severe form, it can lead to the person falling to the floor. These 'attacks' are often prompted by emotion, such as laughing or anger. Sleep paralysis is body paralysis whilst still being conscious, usually upon waking or going off to sleep. Although uncommon, occasionally someone with narcolepsy will have these experiences on an almost daily basis. Hypnagogic hallucinations are hallucinations that usually occur on waking that incorporate visual elements of the surrounding environment (Rechtschaffen and Siegel, 1999). Treatment for narcolepsy is in the form of stimulants and sleep suppressants, the therapist may be able to help with relaxation methods to combat any side effects of stimulatory medication, particularly those techniques that are 'portable', and therefore can be applied to daily living tasks.

Sleep apnoea. This disorder of sleep is relatively common affecting approximately 5% of the general population. Sleep apnoea results from the relaxation of the soft palate (as during sleep) causing the airway to collapse in people who have a narrow airway. Clearly then, oxygen levels start to drop, and as a result, the sleeper briefly awakes to take a characteristic snorting breath, thereby reopening the airway. This can happen many times during the sleep cycle, and clearly disrupts normal sleep, leaving the sufferer often feeling exhausted the next day. In men, severe obstructive sleep apnoea–hypopnoea significantly increases the risk of fatal and non-fatal cardiovascular events. The continuous positive airway pressure (CPAP, a mask of pressurised air) treatment reduces this risk (Gangswich *et al.*, 2006; Wiernsperger *et al.*, 2006).

Insomnia can occur co-morbidly with a number of mental and physical disorders, but should be classified as a separate disorder if it is a dominant feature and is unrelated to other obvious factors such as shift work (WHO, 1992; Asnis *et al.*, 1999). Severity is measured in accordance with daytime effects on functioning in daily life activities, sleepiness, and negative effects on mood. Two of the most significant types of sleep disorders are narcolepsy and sleep apnoea (see Box 6.1). Insomnia should be easy to detect following examination of a week-long sleep diary.

Sleep management

There are a limited number of studies which specifically examine the underlying lifestyle factors which influence sleep, and which sleep in its turn, hampers (Krystal, 2007). However, non-medication strategies are proving effective with lifestyle factors having the added benefit of being applicable to general health promotion/illness prevention programmes. In any case of sleep disorder, lifestyle advice supported by a sleep diary would be useful. These can be used either in collaboration with medication or specialist advice, or as a lead up to specialist intervention. This process can serve to empower the individual who may be anxious regarding the poor sleep effects and wish to pursue a non-pharmacological solution.

People with insomnia consult and use health care services more frequently than those without a sleep problem (Zammit, 2007). This suggests that a multitude of factors either influence or are influenced by a lack of quality sleep. To suggest that everyone who has difficulties sleeping requires medication would be at best naive, at worst we risk becoming complicit in the client's avoidance of the underlying issues surrounding the sleep disorder. It is with some caution that sleep should be approached as the primary disorder (Morin *et al.*, 2007). It is more important to establish each individual's history of their current life (not just medical history) to elicit whether there is a fundamental issue that is influencing sleep (Summers *et al.*, 2006). A holistic approach needs to be applied to gain resolution of chronic sleep problems, especially where there are demonstrable effects of sleep deprivation (Murphy and Delanty, 2007).

Pharmacological treatments for insomnia

It has been recognised that although pharmacological strategies are most frequently used with sleep problems, careful assessment of the underlying cause for sleep disorder is recommended as well as aiming to prescribe sedating medications for short duration only (Morin *et al.*, 2007). Benzodiazepine use is associated with an increase in sleep duration, but is countered by a number of adverse effects, such as, memory impairment, daytime drowsiness and dizziness (Poyares *et al.*, 1997). These inevitably can interfere with daily life activities and occupational fulfilment and enjoyment (Holbrook *et al.*, 2000). Other than medical practitioners, most health care professionals will have little involvement in the prescription of medicines to help aid sleep. However, it is possible that a number of clients with a variety of disorders, may be taking a pharmacological sleep treatment, which may require support in withdrawal. Side effects of other medications for co-existing conditions (such as diuretics) could interfere with sleep, and it is therefore prudent to enquire about all medications, prescribed or non-prescribed to ascertain if these can inhibit sleep.

Complementary and alternative treatment for insomnia

It has been reported in a large sample of US general adult population with a sleep problem that 4.5% use complementary or alternative medicine (Pearson *et al.*, 2006). Non-prescription over-the-counter sleep remedies, for example, herbs (such as Valerian, St John's Wort) and vitamins are increasingly popular, however, they are uncontrolled and there is little evidence of their efficacy and safety (Pillitteri *et al.*, 1994; Meolie *et al.*, 2005).

Non-pharmacological approaches to sleep management

One of the overarching advantages of using a non-pharmacological route to better sleep is that the poor sleeper assumes greater control of their lives. In addition, the effects are typically longer term, and with minimal negative side effects compared with drug therapies (Ringdahl *et al.*, 2004). Cognitive behavioural strategies such as sleep diaries, strategies to challenge negative or catastrophic thinking in relation to sleep and reduction of daytime sleeps have been found to be particularly effective (Montgomery and Dennis, 2003). Some studies have suggested that long-term CBT, is superior and more effective than that of a pharmacological treatment (Sivertsen *et al.*, 2006).

Examples of behavioural interventions include helping patients to modify maladaptive sleep habits and educating them about healthier sleep practices and routines. However, there is a lack of consensus as to what constitutes sleep 'hygiene' rules (Stepanski and Wyatt, 2003) suggesting that sleep hygiene needs to be within a multicomponent regimen, with cognitive behavioural strategies working in tandem with short-term sleep-inducing medications (Morgenthaler *et al.*, 2006). Modifying sleep behaviours has been found to be helpful in more problematic sleep disorders such as sleep apnoea (Bahia *et al.*, 2006).

Sleep diaries

Over 10 years ago, Pilcher *et al.* (1997) suggested that the link between sleep and health status (such as subjective measures of well-being) was more closely related to sleep quality rather than quantity. The distinction supports recommendations to focus on quality, rather than long hours of sleep. This can be achieved through education of how sleep effects body and mind and what is influencing sleep through examining individual sleep diaries (Advice box 6.1 and Handout 6.1).

A sleep diary allows not only the professional to view the extent of the sleep problem, but also to allow the client to gain a more factual rather than *perceived* extent of the problem. There are comprehensive sleep diaries, such as the 'Pittsburgh sleep diary' (Monk *et al.*, 1994) or using the 'Insomnia Intake History' (Summers *et al.*, 2006, p. 280), all of which are useful in examining the behaviours and cognitions behind the sleep pattern. However, diaries that are brief and easy to complete can produce records of more days while still allowing the client to recognise that they are getting *some* sleep. It is helpful to talk the client through their fears about the effects of lack of sleep ('I'm really forgetful', 'I never have any energy') such black and white statements may arise from a sense of poor self-esteem, depression, or point to a problem in their wider lives, for example, relationships.

Sleep hygiene

Hauri in 1977 created a set of rules based on clinical experience and research of the time and named these 'sleep hygiene' although he now confesses that he was never keen on the title! (Hauri, 1991). These broadly common-sense 'rules' for better sleep are expanded on in Handout 6.3.

Sleep routines and habits

The support for a list of routines often is little more than common sense. However, one study of older adults (Cohen-Mansfield and Jensen, 2005), found that even with sleep compromising illness, those following helpful bed-time routines, for example, regular bedtime, soothing music, bath and lack of stimuli reported better sleep than those who did not. Where daily activities have been measured, there is evidence that greater variability in routine correlated with more disturbed sleep (Carney *et al.*, 2006). Daytime sleeping can interfere with sleep quality at night as well as with daily occupational balance. Hauri talks of 'sleep curtailment' (Hauri, 1991, p. 66), suggesting that sleep quality can be improved if it is taken all at once, with no more than the average amount of time spent in bed. There is evidence that certain major mental illnesses are helped by maintaining a regular sleep–wake routine (Ellen *et al.*, 2006). It is unsurprising, therefore, that shift work which ultimately confounds the body's circadian rhythm with changes to daily and nightly routines has been associated with sleep-related symptomology. Large-scale studies such as that by Drake *et al.* (2004) suggest that shift workers are at significant risk of behavioural and health-related morbidity. A well-written and easily obtainable leaflet illustrating 'healthy sleep routines' is produced by the Royal College of Psychiatrists and is downloadable for client use (Royal College of Psychiatrists, 2005), however, a comprehensive guide is also supplied in Handout 6.2, with advice to promote change in Advice Box 6.2.

Exercise and sleep

Although studies recommend that light to moderate exercise (such as brisk walking or low-impact aerobics) can improve self-reported quality of sleep in older (King *et al.*, 1997) and working age (Atlantis *et al.*, 2006) adults (especially when taken early evening, i.e. not just prior to going to bed), a meta-analysis of the effects of exercise on sleep suggests that there is room for further exploration (Youngstedt *et al.*, 1997). Possibly because there is evidence that where individuals are sleep deprived, moderate exercise makes them more vulnerable to mood disturbance and reduces reaction times, which in turn can increase the risk of accidents (Scott *et al.*, 2006). Current health promotion (DH, 2005) encourages healthy subjects to engage in moderate exercise. Where local government initiatives have been used, it has been measured as being cost-effective in terms of cost of ill-health versus cost of implementing exercise programmes (DH, 2007). The link between hypertension and short-sleep duration is a point of case, exercise can effectively resolve two problems at the same time, incorporating exercise regularly can decrease blood pressure, and in turn improve sleep quality (Gangwisch *et al.*, 2006). By introducing exercise within contexts during the day into general routines of daily life (e.g. if working in high-rise offices, taking the stairs several times in the day) individuals may be more compliant and motivated to be more active, especially in subjects who consider exercise is a meaningless 'chore' and not an occupation of choice.

Eating, drinking, smoking and sleep

Nearly 25% of young men profess to using alcohol to induce sleep (Pillitteri *et al.*, 1994); yet, despite findings suggesting that alcohol consumption is associated with longer time spent in bed, it is also associated with less restorative sleep, ultimately reducing the quality (Lauderdale *et al.*, 2006). Increased levels of anxiety are associated with smoking (Ulrich *et al.*, 2004) which is also (due to the stimulatory effects of nicotine) a factor in causing difficulty falling and staying asleep (Htoo *et al*, 2004; Lauderdale *et al.*, 2006). Drinking fluids just prior to bed may have an inhibitory effect on sleep, not just in terms of stimulants such as caffeine. A trip to the bathroom may be frustratingly part of life, but it may be as a result of the milky drink before bedtime.

Old wives' tales suggest that eating before bedtime can influence dreams and sleep (i.e. cheese causing bad dreams), however, perhaps it is the point of when one eats. It is quite often the case, that heartburn/reflux, and so on, occurs at night. Lying prone whilst digesting food is not recommended for quality sleep.

Adapting daily occupations

Chronic insomnia or rather the chronic effects of a lack of sleep can reduce occupational performance particularly in cognitive concentrative tasks (Wlodarczyk *et al.*, 2002). If cognitive skills are deleteriously affected due to sleep deprivation, occupational performance may be improved by grading activities and occupations, for example, by incorporating frequent breaks, performing complex tasks at the most alert time of day, and gradually building up ability where a task is newly learnt. Keeping lists, setting time limits for tasks and ensuring the environment for working is not distracting can also help enhance concentration. There is evidence that television watching and using computer games to aid sleep can reduce quality and quantity of sleep (Johnson *et al.*, 2004; Eggermont and Van den Bulck, 2006). Environmental noise, such as traffic, interferes with perceived quality and quantity of sleep in adults (Öhrström *et al.*, 2006).

Being frequently unable to do what you want to do can result in a reduction in self-esteem, confidence and empowerment (Hasselkus, 2002). Adjustments to lifestyle, engaging in differing occupations, including increasing social support, and reducing work demands are recommended to reduce disturbed sleep (Akerstedt *et al.*, 2002). Boredom and meaningless occupation reduce motivation and performance thereby inducing daytime sleepiness and inattention (Kass *et al.*, 2003). By engaging in relaxing, enjoyable and meaningful occupations of choice within a habitual routine can benefit health (Law *et al.*, 1998; Montgomery and Dennis, 2002)and as a result, improve sleep.

Cognitive approaches to sleep management

It has been established that individuals can exaggerate the extent of their sleep problem (Morin, 1993; Harvey, 2002; Summers *et al.*, 2006). However, it is suggested that sleep monitors, when compared to self-reported sleep diaries, show a reduction in the overall anxiety about the lack of sleep, and a corresponding effect on levels of insomnia (Tang and Harvey, 2004). A similar approach of completing diaries by the bed (not completed too retrospectively post-sleep), and explored with therapists to establish the scale of disruption compared to normal sleep, can be helpful. Intrusive thoughts and worrying can particularly cause difficulties in getting to sleep (Morin, 1993), this can be modified by utilising cognitive methods to either challenge the worrying thought with facts or by writing down the thoughts which allows the mind to 'let go' of the need to ruminate. There is a tendency for people with chronic insomnia to retire to bed with anticipatory anxiety of another sleepless night, thus triggering arousal and thus leading to the inevitable difficulty in falling asleep (Harvey, 2002; Summers *et al.*, 2006). This may be helped by using mantras of positive thoughts such as 'Tonight I will sleep well' or using a strategy such as the mantra technique suggested in Chapter 7.

Other strategies may involve helping the individual to recognise when they use 'catastrophic' or exaggerated thinking such as 'I've not slept all week', which is very unlikely to be the case.

Conclusion

Sleep problems can lead to frequent health utilisation, particularly in women, whereas men tend to use alcohol to procure night-time sleep. There can be an underlying illness influencing sleep, and insomnia can be a troublesome symptom in a number of disorders. There are a number of lifestyle factors contributing to poor sleep, and a number of physical- and mental-health-related problems associated with, or which cause, insomnia. Although modern medications have fewer side effects and less withdrawal effects than those of the past, it is still the adoption of certain lifestyle behaviours that provide the best long-term solution to non-organic insomnia problems.

There are increasing amounts of studies that include simple sleep advice/routine as a mainstay in the treatment of chronic insomnia, these can be superior to that of prescribed medication that take the locus of control from the client, and could obscure the underlying reason for the sleep problem. A sleep diary pre- and post-sleep advice/routines allows for a realistic overview of the sleep problem at hand, as there is often a tendency to over-exaggerate the extent of the sleep problem. By sharing facts about sleep and following basic behavioural goals within a habitual routine, the sleep problem can be managed and overcome. In encouraging a daily lifestyle with some exercise and meaningful and not overtly stimulatory activity prior to sleep, the focus of attention is diverted from the anxiety associated with insomnia.

In providing a range of strategies, evidence-based advice and handout information, this chapter has aimed to offer the health and social care professional; a comprehensive package to facilitate control of the sleep problem, break lifestyle habits inhibiting sleep, and adopt routines that empower the client/patient. Left with no intervention at all, the problem of insomnia and resultant sleep deprivation can lead to anxiety disorders and accidents through poor concentration with potential disastrous consequences.

References

Akerstedt, T. and Nilsson, P. M. (2003). Sleep as restitution: an introduction. *Journal of Internal Medicine*, 254: 6–12.

Akerstedt, T., Knutsson, A., Westerholm, P., Theorell, T., Alfredsson, L. and Kecklund, G. (2002). Sleep disturbances, work stress and work hours: a cross-sectional study. *Journal of Psychosomatic Research*, 53(3): 741–748.

American Academy of Sleep Medicine (2005). *ICSD – International Classification of Sleep Disorders, Revised: Diagnostic and Coding Manual.* American Academy of Sleep Medicine, Westchester, IL.

Asnis, G. M., Chakraburtty, A. and DuBoff, E. A. (1999). Zolpidem in SSRI-treated patients with persistent insomnia. *Journal of Clinical Psychiatry*, 60: 668–676.

Atlantis, E., Chow, C. M., Kirby, A. and Fiatarone Singh, M. (2006). Worksite intervention effects on sleep quality: a randomized controlled trial. *Journal of Occupational Health Psychology*, 11(4): 291–304.

Bahia, G., Soares, A. V. and Winck, C. J. (2006). Impact of sleep hygiene on patients with obstructive sleep apnoea syndrome. *Revista Portuguesa de Pneumologia*, 12(2): 147–176.

Bonnet, M. H. and Arand, D. L. (1995). We are chronically sleep deprived. *Sleep*, 18(10): 908–911.

Carmona, R. H. (2004). Introductory remarks, frontiers of knowledge in sleep and sleep disorders: opportunities for improving health and quality of life. *Journal of Clinical Sleep Medicine*, 1: 83–85.

Carney, R. M., Howells, W. B., Freedland, K. E. *et al.* (2006). Depression and obstructive sleep apnea in patients with coronary heart disease. *Psychosomatic Medicine*, 68: 443–448.

Carskdon, M. A. and Dement, W. C. (2000). Normal human sleep: an overview. In Kryger, M. H., Roth, T. and Dement, W. C. (eds) *Principles and Practice of Sleep Medicine*, 3rd edition. Philadelphia, PA, W. B. Saunders, pp. 15–25.

Chasens, E. R. (2007). Understanding sleep in persons with diabetes. *The Diabetes Educator*, 33(3): 435–436.

Cohen-Mansfield, J. and Jensen, B. (2005). Sleep-related habits and preferences in older adults: a pilot study of their range and self-rated importance. *Behavioral Sleep Medicine*, 3(4): 209–226.

Davidson, J. R., MacLean, A. W., Brundage, M. D. and Schulze, K. (2002). Sleep disturbance in cancer patients. *Social Science & Medicine*, 54(9): 1309–1321.

DH (2005). *Choosing Activity: A Physical Activity Action Plan*. London, Department of Health.

DH (2007). *LEAP. Local Exercise Action Pilots.* London, Department of Health.

Drake, C., Roehrs, T., Richardson, G., Walsh, J. K. and Roth, T. (2004). Shift work sleep disorder: prevalence and consequences beyond that of symptomatic day workers. *Sleep*, 27(8): 1453–1462.

Eggermont, S. and Van den Bulck, J. (2006). Nodding off or switching off? The use of popular media as a sleep aid in secondary-school children. *Journal of Paediatrics and Child Health*, 42(7–8): 428–433.

Ellen, F., Gonzalez, J. M. and Fagiolini, A. (2006). The importance of routine for preventing recurrence in bipolar disorder. *American Journal of Psychiatry*, 163: 981–985.

Gangwisch, J. E., Heymsfield, S. B., Boden-Albala, B. *et al.* (2006). Short sleep duration as a risk factor for hypertension analyses of the first national health and nutrition examination survey. *Hypertension*, 47: 833.

Greene, R. and Siegel, J. (2004). *Sleep: A Functional Enigma NeuroMolecular Medicine*, Humana Press, New Jersey, vol. 5, no. 1, pp. 59–68.

Groeger, J. A., Zijlstra, F. R. H. and Dijk, D. J. (2004). Sleep quantity, sleep difficulties and their perceived consequences in a representative sample of some 2000 British adults. *Journal of Sleep Research*, 13(4): 359–371.

Harvey, A. G. (2002). A cognitive model of insomnia. *Behaviour Research and Therapy*, 40: 869–893.

Hasselkus, B. R. (2002). *The Meaning of Everyday Occupation*. Thorofare, NJ, SLACK Inc.

Hauri, P. J. (1991). Sleep hygiene, relaxation therapy and cognitive interventions. In Hauri, P. J. (ed.) *Case Studies in Insomnia*. New York, Plenum Press, pp. 1–15.

Holbrook, A. M., Crowther, R., Lotter, A., Cheng, C. and King, D. (2000). Meta-analysis of benzodiazepine use in the treatment of insomnia. *CMAJ*, 162(2): 225–233.

Htoo, A., Talwar, A. and Feinsilver, S. H. (2004). Smoking and sleep disorders. *Medical Clinics of North America*, 88: 1575–1591.

Johnson, J. G., Cohen, P., Kasen, S., First, M. B. and Brook, J. S. (2004). Association between television viewing and sleep problems during adolescence and early adulthood. *Archives of Pediatrics & Adolescent Medicine*, 158: 562–568.

Kass, Steven J., Wallace, J. Craig and Vodanovich, Stephen J. (2003). Boredom proneness and sleep disorders as predictors of adult attention deficit scores. *Journal of Attention Disorders*, 7: 83–91.

King, A. C., Oman, R. F., Brassington, G. S., Bliwise, D. L. and Haskell, W. L. (1997). Moderate-intensity exercise and self-rated quality of sleep in older adults. A randomized controlled trial. *Journal of American Medical Association*, 277(1): 32–37.

Kronholm, E., Härmä, M., Hublin, C., Aro, A. R. and Partonen, T. (2006). Self-reported sleep duration in Finnish general population. *Journal of Sleep Research*, 15(3): 276–290.

Krystal, A. D. (2007). Treating the health, quality of life, and functional impairments in insomnia. *Journal of Clinical Sleep Medicine: JCSM: Official Publication of the American Academy of Sleep Medicine*, 3(1): 63–72.

Lauderdale, D. S., Kristen, L. Knutson, Lijing L. Y. *et al.* (2006). Objectively measured sleep characteristics among early-middle-aged adults the CARDIA study. *American Journal of Epidemiology*, 164(1): 5–16.

Law, M., Steinwender, S. and Leclair, L. (1998). Occupation, health and well-being. *Canadian Journal of Occupational Therapy*, 65(2): 81–91.

Marin, S., Carrizo, E. and Agusti, V. A. (2005). Long-term cardiovascular outcomes in men with obstructive sleep apnoea–hypopnoea with or without treatment with continuous positive airway pressure: an observational study. *Lancet*, 365(9464): 1046–1053.

Meolie, A. L., Rosen, C., Kristo, D. *et al.* (2005). Oral non-prescription treatment for insomnia: An evaluation of products with limited evidence. *Journal of Clinical Sleep Medicine*, 1(2): 173–187.

Monk, T. M., Reynolds, C. F., Kupfer, D. J. *et al.* (1994). The Pittsburgh sleep diary. *Journal of Sleep Research*, 3(2): 111–120.

Montgomery, P. and Dennis, J. (2002). Physical exercise for sleep problems in adults aged 60+. *Cochrane Database of Systematic Reviews*, (4), Art. No. CD003404.

Montgomery, P. and Dennis, J. (2003). Cognitive behavioural interventions for sleep problems in adults aged 60+. *Cochrane Database of Systematic Reviews*, (1).

Morgenthaler, T., Kramer, M., Alessi, C. *et al.* (2006). Practice parameters for the psychological and behavioral treatment of insomnia: an update. An American Academy of Sleep Medicine Report. *Sleep*, 29(11): 1415–1419.

Morin, A. K., Jarvis, C. I. and Lynch, A. M. (2007). Therapeutic options for sleep-maintenance and sleep-onset insomnia. *Pharmacotherapy*, 27(1): 89–110.

Morin, C. M. (1993). *Insomnia: Psychological Assessment and Management.* New York, Guildford Press.

Morin, C. M. (2006). Combined therapeutics for insomnia: should our first approach be behavioral or pharmacological? *Sleep Medicine*, 7(1): 15–19.

Morin, C. M., Bootzin, R. R., Buysee, D. J., Edinger, J. D., Espie, C. A. and Lichstein, K. L. (2006). Psychological and behavioral treatment of insomnia: update of the recent evidence (1998–2004). *Sleep*, 29(11): 1398–1414.

Morin, C. M., LeBlanc, M., Daley, M., Gregoire, J. P. and Mérette, C. (2006). Epidemiology of insomnia: prevalence, self-help treatments, consultations, and determinants of help-seeking behaviours. *Sleep Medicine*, 7(2): 123–130.

Murphy, K. and Delanty, N. (2007). Sleep deprivation: a clinical perspective. *Sleep and Biological Rhythms*, 5(1): 2–14.

National Sleep Foundation (2007). *How Sleep Works.* Available: http://www.sleepfoundation.org/site/c.huIXKjM0IxF/b.2417141/k.2E30/The_National_Sleep_Foundation.htm. Last accessed 1 September 2007.

Neckelmann, D., Mykletun, A. and Dahl, A. A. (2007). Insomnia as a risk factor for developing anxiety and depression. *Sleep*, 30(7): 873–880.

Neubauer, D. N. (2006). New approaches in managing chronic insomnia. *CNS Spectrums*, 11(8): 1–13.

Öhrström, E., Hadzibajramovic, E., Holmes, M. and Svensson, H. (2006). Effects of road traffic noise on sleep: Studies on children and adults. *Journal of Environment Psychology*, 26(2): 116–126.

Pearson, N. J., Johnson, L. L. and Nahin, R. L. (2006). Insomnia, trouble sleeping, and complementary and alternative medicine. Analysis of the 2002 National Health Interview Survey Data. *Archives of Internal Medicine*, 166: 1775–1782.

Pilcher, J. J., Ginter, D. R. and Sadowsky, B. (1997). Sleep quality versus sleep quantity: Relationships between sleep and measures of health, well-being and sleepiness in college students. *Journal of Psychosomatic Research*, 42(6): 513–514.

Pillitteri, J. L., Kozlowski, L. T., Person, D. C. and Spear, M. E. (1997). Over-the-counter sleep aids: widely used but rarely studied. *Journal of Substance Abuse*, 6(3): 315–323.

Poyares, D., Guilleminault, C., Ohayon, M. M. and Tufik, S. (2004). Chronic benzodiazepine usage and withdrawal in insomnia patients. *Journal of Psychiatric Research*, 38(3): 327–334.

Rechtschaffen, A. and Siegel, J. A. (1999). Sleep and dreaming. In Kandel, E. R., Schwartz, J. H. and Jessell, T. J. (eds) *Principles of Neural Science*, 4th edition. New York, McGraw-Hill.

Reichmuth, K. J., Austin, D. A., Skatrud, J. B. and Young, T. (2005). Association of sleep apnea and type II diabetes: A population-based study. *American Journal of Respiratory and Critical Care Medicine*, 172: 1590–1595.

Ringdahl, E. N., Pereira, S. L. and Delzell, J. E. (2004). Treatment of primary insomnia. *The Journal of the American Board of Family Practice*. 17: 212–219.

Sateia, M. J., Doghramji, K., Hauri, P. J. and Morin., C. M. (2000). Evaluation of chronic insomnia: An American Academy of Sleep Medicine review. *Sleep*, 23: 243–308.

Savage, V. M. and West, G. (2007). A quantitative, theoretical framework for understanding mammalian sleep. *Proceedings of the National Academy of Sciences*, 104(3): 1051–1056.

Scott, J. P., McNaughton, L. R. and Polman, R. C. (2006). Effects of sleep deprivation and exercise on cognitive, motor performance and mood. *Physiology & Behavior*, 87(2): 396–408.

Seicean, A., Redline, S., Seicean, S. *et al.* (2007). Association between short sleeping hours and overweight in adolescents: Results from a US suburban high school survey. *Sleep and Breathing*, 14.

Sivertsen, B., Omvik, S., Pallesen, S. *et al.* (2006). Cognitive behavioral therapy vs zopiclone for treatment of chronic primary insomnia in older adults: A randomized controlled trial. *Journal of American Medical Association*, 295(24): 2851–2858.

Spiegel, K., Knutson, K., Leproult, R., Tasali, E. and van Cauter, E. (2005). Sleep loss: A novel risk factor for insulin resistance and type 2 diabetes. *Journal of Applied Physiology*, 99: 2008–2019.

Stepanski, E. J. and Wyatt, J. K. (2003). Use of sleep hygiene in the treatment of insomnia. *Sleep Medicine Reviews*, 7(3): 213–225.

Stremler, R., Hodnett, E., Lee, K. *et al.* (2006). A behavioral–educational intervention to promote maternal and infant sleep: A pilot randomized, controlled trial. *Sleep*, 29(12): 1609–1615.

Suka, M., Yoshida, K. and Sugimori, H. (2003). Persistent insomnia is a predictor of hypertension in Japanese male workers. *Journal of Occupational Health*, 45(6): 344–350.

Summers, M. O., Crisostomo, M. I. and Stepanski, E. J. (2006). Recent developments in the classification, evaluation, and treatment of insomnia. *Chest*, 130: 276–286.

Tang, N. K. Y. and Harvey, A. G. (2004). Correcting distorted perception of sleep: A novel treatment component for insomnia? *Behaviour Research and Therapy*, 42(1): 27–39.

Ulrich, J., Meyer, C., Rumpf, H. -J. and Hapke, U. (2004). Smoking, nicotine dependence and psychiatric comorbidity – a population-based study including smoking cessation after three years. *Drug and Alcohol Dependence*, 76(3): 287–295.

Van Dongen, H. P., Maislin, G., Mullington, J. M. and Dinges, D. F. (2003). The cumulative cost of additional wakefulness: Dose–response effects on neurobehavioral functions and sleep physiology from chronic sleep restriction and total sleep deprivation. *Sleep*, 26(2): 117–126.

Vgontzas, A. N. and Kales, A. (1999). Sleep and its disorders. *Annual Review of Medicine*, 50: 387–400.

Walsleben, J. A., Kapur, V. K., Newman, A. B. *et al.* (2004). Sleep and reported daytime sleepiness in normal subjects: The sleep heart health study. *Sleep*, 27: 293–298.

Wiernsperger, N., Nivoit, P. and Bouskela, E. (2006). Obstructive sleep apnea and insulin resistance: a role for microcirculation? *Clinics* [serial on the Internet]. June [cited 21 August 2007], 61(3): 253–266. http://www.scielo.br/scielo.php?script=sci_arttext&pid=S1807-59322006000300011&lng=en&nrm=iso

Wlodarczyk, D., Jaskowski, P. and Nowik, A. (2002). Influence of sleep deprivation and auditory intensity on reaction time and response force. *Perceptual and Motor Skills*, 94: 101–112.

WHO (1992). *International Statistical Classification of Disease and Related Health Problems, Tenth Revision (ICD-10)*. Geneva, World Health Organization.

Youngstedt, S. D., O'Connor, P. J. and Dishman, R. K. (1997). The effects of acute exercise on sleep: A quantitative synthesis. *Sleep*, 20(3): 203–214.

Zammit, G. K. (2007). The prevalence, morbidities, and treatments of insomnia. *CNS & Neurological Disorders Drug Targets*, 6(1), 3–16.

Zammit, G. K., Weiner, J., Damato, N., Sillup, G. P. and McMillan, C. A. (1999). Quality of life in people with insomnia. *Insomnia: Sleep*, 22 (suppl 2): S379–S385.

Further reading

Hauri, P. (1977). *Current Concepts: The Sleep Disorders*. Kalamazoo, MI, The Upjohn Company.

Shneerson, J. (2005). *Sleep Medicine: A Guide to Sleep and Its Disorders*. Oxford, Blackwell Publishing.

Useful books/resources

www.sleepfoundation.org
www.nnt.nhs.uk/mh/leaflets/sleep%20problems%20a5.pdf
www.helpguide.org/life/sleep_disorders.htm
Royal College of Psychiatrists (2005). *Sleeping Well*. Royal College of Psychiatrists. London. http://www.rcpsych.ac.uk/mentalhealthinformation/mentalhealthproblems/sleepproblems/sleepingwell.aspx. Retrieved 25 May 2007.

All of the following handouts and advice boxes can be found as individual pdfs on the website at www.blackwellpublishing.com/thew

Advice box 6.1 Using the sleep diary (Handout 6.1)

The client will have to have completed the sleep diary for one total week (two ideally) and this needs to be a 'typical' week (not during an un-typical time like a holiday), enquire if the individual has noticed any patterns or causes for their problems.

Analyse the diary. For example, which night/s of the week was the sleep particularly bad? Ask what had been happening during the day; enquire regarding any specific worries, sleep may not be the primary problem, if there is a relationship, work or other problems, explanation of how these may interfere with sleep may be prudent, rather than focusing on the sleep problem alone.

The more attention someone attaches to the sleep problem, the more watchful and anxious one can become leading to an exacerbation of insomnia. It may therefore be only necessary to view the sleep diary and reassure the client that their sleep is 'normal' in terms of the population average. It may also be clear that there are routine, environmental and other factors that are likely to be causing the problem; talk the client through each point of the handouts, for example, reinforce the importance of routine, and cut out any daytime naps, and so on. Handout 6.2 provides some information on what 'normal' sleep is to help reassure the client. Teaching relaxation strategies can be helpful in addressing the sleep problem as well as the 'daytime' problems.

Keeping another sleep diary post 2 weeks of following advice and routines allows for comparison. If there is no change to the quality/quantity of sleep, it may be worth exploring with the individual's general practitioner whether short-term medication alongside the advice would be useful, the advice can then be maintained after the prescription expires.

Advice box 6.2 Establishing routines

It may be difficult to motivate an individual to stick to a routine, especially if they are taking daytime naps, and enjoying them! It would only be helpful if there is a healthy amount of activity and stimulation during the day, with late night rest prior to going to bed to sleep. NB: Falling asleep on the sofa in the early evening should be classed as 'daytime' sleep. Establish what would be gained from having no daytime naps (e.g. what occupations would be possible), how do they feel after the nap?

Some individuals can argue that they sleep in until midday because they are 'night-owls', and 'can't' get to sleep until the early hours. This can be challenged by using an example of how the body reacts to different time zones whilst on holiday: for example, the body will adjust to the daylight hours, and sleep during the night-time, however, whilst the body is adjusting, the sensation is that of 'jet-lag'!

Present the evidence on how the body performs better following a routine, and how sleep is often of better quality if taken within a shorter period of time.

Set a definite bedtime and wake-up time, this has to become a habit and therefore needs to be followed everyday of the week, no matter how the person feels, acknowledge that this may initially be a struggle, however, like a long haul holiday, the body clock will adjust. It may require a desensitisation approach to reducing the hours spent awake in the middle of the night, by making the body more 'greedy' for sleep, by getting up much earlier than usual, by forcing the body to stay alert all day and by going to bed at the usual time, thus causing deep sleep to be taken in the middle of the night.

If there is a desire to sleep during the day, then expectation of good sleep at night has to be lowered. Note if there is frequent waking in the night: ascertain if these are due to frequent trips to the loo – the eating and drinking habits may need addressing. It may be helpful to ascertain if any medications (such as diuretics) are causing night-time disturbances.

If there is difficulty getting off to sleep, suggest strategies of relaxation, or engaging in sedentary meaningful occupations but avoiding watching emotive television, and computer activities prior to sleep.

If the diary shows evidence of an overtly sedentary lifestyle during the day with copious hours resting (not sleeping) suggest reducing the hours at rest and increasing (via grading up) light or moderate exercise, or engaging in occupations that require the body to be active.

Handout 6.1 Sleep diary

					Week commencing:		
Instructions: complete boxes 1–2 prior to retiring for the night, complete boxes 3–5 in the morning (when wake up….)							
Day of week	**Monday**	**Tuesday**	**Wednesday**	**Thursday**	**Friday**	**Saturday**	**Sunday**
What did you do today?							
How sleepy did you feel today?/No. of naps							
Time you went to bed							
Time it took to fall asleep (minutes)							
How many times did you wake up?							
Quality of sleep (0–5)[a]							
Total hours asleep:							

[a] 0 = Very poor, 1 = Poor, 2 = average, 3 = good, 4 = very good, 5 = excellent.

Handout 6.2 Sleep – The life enhancer

Sleep affects all that we do, we crave 'perfect' sleep, and can feel very low if we are sleep deprived even for only one night. Many things influence the quantity and quality of sleep. We are all individuals, and we all know someone who is a 'bad' sleeper. More often than not, it is a temporary 'bad' sleep that we suffer. Sometimes, however, it can be more prolonged, thus needing some help.

Analyse your sleep. Sometime there is a simple reason why your sleep is not so good at the moment, for example, being nervous about something (even good things, such as getting married!). This is normal, and you may just need to try to deal with the problem rather than worrying about it! By completing a sleep diary for at least one complete week and then looking at it, you may find that there are some obvious reasons for your sleep that you had not realised.

What to look out for

How many hours, on average, have you slept over the entire week? You may find that some nights you get much less than the general population (which is between 6 and 8 hours a night) and other nights you are compensating by sleeping for longer. The average time in quality (restorative) sleep is about 6½ hours. Women tend to sleep longer than men, and generally, the younger you are the more sleep you tend to take. However, most people tend to sleep for longer than is necessary.

What did you eat/do/drink the day before? This can have significant effects on the quality of your sleep, drinking alcohol, for example, may make you fall asleep, but the quality of sleep is poor, often you will notice that you feel very tired the day after a dinking session! Eating just before bedtime can also affect your sleep, partly because lying down can make the acid in your stomach to reflux, causing pain.

Are you overactive just before bed time? If you are very active, this can help sleep, but if you are over stimulated just before going to bed it can over stimulate you and sleep is harder to obtain.

Are you lying awake thinking and worrying? Stress can influence your sleep, and it can be a case of worry keeping you awake. Then you worry about not being able to sleep, which causes the circle of worry/sleeplessness going round and round.

Handout 6.2 Continued

Are you lying in bed dozing for hours and hours but awaken still feeling tired? Sleep that is good quality is more important than sleep that is of long duration, but is spread out over a long period of time. That is why sleep programmes actually restrict the amount you sleep, in order to increase its quality.

Are you thinking the problem is worse than it really is? Many sleep studies have found that people often think they have slept less than they really have, be realistic about how much sleep you need, you may actually NEED less than you think!

Handout 6.3 Sleep management principles

There are a number of self-help strategies which may well be worth trying before resorting to taking prescription medicine or even herbal or alternative medicine – which can be costly and make you feel tired the next day. All of the tips below are based on research and are not 'old wives' tales. They may seem common sense, but often we do not practice common sense in our daily lives!

Follow the advice below for 2 weeks and use the sleep diary to monitor progress

1. *Go to bed and get up at more or less the exact same time every day.* This will get your body clock into a rhythm. Routines are really helpful for sleep problems, if you have ever had children you will know how important routine.
2. *As part of the bedtime routine, incorporate a warm bath, after a sedentary occupation/hobby.* Avoid stimulatory tasks such as playing computer games or working or exercising – this can keep you awake.
3. Eat proper meals and drink plenty during the day and into the evening time, avoiding eating or drinking an hour before bedtime. This will prevent the night-time trip to the loo, or reduce the likelihood of indigestion.
4. *Do not use alcohol to aid sleep.* It may make you feel tired, but actually it is making the quality of your sleep worse, and you can wake up feeling un-refreshed.
5. *Do not smoke just before bedtime.* Even nicotine can have a stimulatory effect, try and avoid this in the evening.
6. *Ideally, your bedroom environment needs to be conducive for sleep.* Quiet, dark, warm (not hot) temperature, firm, but not overly hard mattress.
7. *If you wake in the night, getting up* rather than tossing and turning may help, as long as you do not engage in stimulatory occupations.
8. *Try writing down worrying thoughts/or task list for the next day* rather than lying there worrying about remembering what you need to do the next day!

Handout 6.3 Continued

9. *Repeating to yourself mentally 'I am going to have a good night's sleep tonight'* over and over again can block out intrusive thoughts, and set your mind onto a positive track.
10. *Light exercise in the day (not late at night)* has been found to help aid sleep. A brisk walk at lunchtimes, or just taking the stairs all the time at work could be included into your daily routine.

Useful resources and websites

The Royal College of Psychiatrists have produced a helpful leaflet including advice on some specific sleep disorders: www.rcpsych.ac.uk/pdf/sleep.pdf

National Sleep Foundation is also helpful: www.sleepfoundation.org

7. *Portable Relaxation for Everyday Living*

Miranda Thew

Introduction

Stress and anxiety represent a global health problem. In Britain work-related stress, depression or anxiety account for an estimated 10.5 million lost working days per year (HSE, 2007). Relaxation techniques have been widely used for many years for the treatment of physical, mental and emotional effects that arise from stress, depression and anxiety. However, in many health-related consultations, the role of psychosocial factors are often overlooked in favour of more formal 'medical' interventions such as prescribed medications. This chapter focusses on the biopsychosocial model which endorses mind–body interventions.

A wide variety of relaxation techniques can be employed to manage anxiety or stress and these techniques can be more effective than listening to soothing music or closing the eyes in a quiet room (Jacobs and Friedman, 2004). Many have involved single- or multicomponent treatments, and although there are useful, and accessible web-based evidence databases, such as OTseeker for occupational therapists (McKenna *et al.*, 2004), there is still a need for the evidence to be condensed and presented, in a suitable, practical and applicable manner to suit the needs of staff in different clinical settings and to increase therapists' confidence to apply knowledge and skills (McCluskey, 2003). Indeed, many techniques of relaxation involve following detailed instructions in manufactured relaxed environments which make them impractical for daily life and too demanding for integration into practical routines. While it must be acknowledged that more 'complete' delivery approaches may house additional beneficial effects, this chapter is concerned with relaxation techniques that can be easily integrated into everyday routines. The relevant stategies presented in this chapter are frequently used within stress management programmes or have been anecdotally popular in my clinical career, which spans two decades. The recommended relaxation strategies can be quickly taught, easily learned and are adaptable to most occupations of life. Underpinning the handouts and techniques is (1) current research regarding their efficacy with a variety of health and well-being settings and (2) evidence to support their clinical application.

Effects of relaxation on health and well-being

Overall, there is strong evidence that relaxation, or rather a relaxed lifestyle, has proven benefits for many health-related problems. It is highly likely that most health and social care professionals will be encountering people whose illness or problems are caused or made worse by stress symptoms. It is, therefore, prudent to be proficient in teaching some useful, applicable stress management techniques that will suit most clients.

There has been criticism that the integration of the mind with the body is so profound that any health care that separates the physiological from the psychological concerns may be unwise (McNair *et al.*, 2002). Indeed, many physical conditions are co-morbidly associated with mental health disorders (Kessler *et al.*, 2002). In anxiety and depression, these associations are thought to be partly due to lifestyle behaviours (Sobel and Markov, 2005). Psychosocial stress is the opposite of relaxation which is known to contribute to high blood pressure and subsequent cardiovascular morbidity and mortality. Anxiety disorders are associated with decreased performance in life occupations and quality of life, and with increased days off work. For this reason, there is a strong recommendation to address anxiety problems in primary care settings (Stein *et al.*, 2005; Greenstone, 2007). Lambert *et al.* (2007) suggest that a lifestyle approach may help general practitioners (GPs) to address anxiety as effectively as routine care. In Australia, a nationally funded programme for primary care providers is based on a three-step programme that engages the client at primary care level directly into receiving or accessing psychological help, including non-pharmacological strategies (Hickie and Groom, 2002). This has been established as cost-effective and is aimed to be preventive. Where panic disorder was treated using a brief primary care cognitive/relaxation intervention, outcomes highlighted that the intervention was not only feasible, but also significantly more effective than usual care (Roy-Byrne *et al.*, 2005).

Stress and depression in the workplace has become a focus of the Health and Safety Executive (HSE) with 10.5 million working days lost each year (HSE, 2007). It is now increasingly common that organisations are providing work-based programmes to tackle the stress 'epidemic' (Palmer *et al.*, 2004; Gyllensten and Palmer, 2005), with good effects not just on stress levels but also on depression/mood states (Shamini, *et al.*, 2007; Mino *et al.*, 2006).

A yoga-based lifestyle has been found to have significant benefits for coronary heart disease symptoms (Yogendra *et al.*, 2004). However, critics of 'relaxation alone' suggest that, as in the case of fibromyalgia patients, long-term effects may be more attributable to the self-efficacy elements of mind–body therapies, that is, benefits result from the patients' belief that they can control a challenging situation (Hadhazy *et al.*, 2000). A systematic review of the effects of relaxation therapy on ischemic heart disease found that not only was relaxation effective in enhancing recovery from heart attack, but it was also instrumental in controlling resting heart rate; resting heart rate also ameliorated the effects of angina thereby reducing mortality and increased return to work (Van Dixhoorn and White, 2005). Hypertension is a major burden on health care, there is evidence that relaxation methods can reduce blood pressure by an average of 10 mm Hg – systolic and 5 mm Hg – diastolic (Astin *et al.*, 2003). Another study with systemically hypertensive older adults suggests that stress-decreasing interventions may contribute to decreased mortality from cardiovascular disease (Schneider *et al.*, 2005). Incorporating daily stress-reduction strategies along with exercise and healthy eating is also recommended to reduce the risk of coronary heart disease (Daubenmeir *et al.*, 2007).

There is such an association between pain and anxiety/tension that many pain management programmes now include relaxation techniques (Persson *et al.*, 2004; Budh *et al.*, 2006). One systematic review of relaxation training with cancer patients found that symptoms improved with intervention, suggesting that it should be implemented in clinical routines (Luebbert *et al.*, 2001). In a different study, women identified stress as the principal cause for their breast cancer – above diet, genetics and other factors (Stewart *et al.*, 2001) – suggesting that they will respond positively to appropriate programme content. Multidisciplinary teams involved in palliative and oncology care, frequently incorporate relaxation within their treatment programmes (Hindley and Johnston, 1999; Vockins, 2004), to reduce anxiety, (Carlson *et al.*, 2003) offer a sense of control, alleviate pain and to also address issues of breathlessness (Ewer-Smith and Patterson, 2002; Vockins, 2004). Further, people with pain are more susceptible to depression, and those with depression are more likely to report being in pain. Given that somatic symptoms, pain and depression are intertwined, the potential value of pain-reducing interventions are clearly advocated.

The National Institute for Clinical Excellence (NICE) guidelines (NICE, 2007) suggest that anxiety and panic disorders are best addressed through a cognitive behavioural approach that includes relaxation techniques; advice, and self-help, alternative treatments are also recommended. However, critics of teaching 'simple' techniques such as diaphragmatic breathing alone, question the value of the 'quick fix' which provides a false sense of safety. Therefore, in the first instance, individuals with a significant anxiety disorder should be referred to a cognitive behavioural therapy trained professional (Roy-Byrne *et al.*, 2005). However, there are fundamental issues of training costs and time, which could prohibit meeting the appropriate NICE guidelines for primary care (Layard, 2006).

Relaxation, either in combination with a cognitive behavioural approach or as a stand-alone intervention, benefits a multitude of physical (Thomas *et al.*, 2003; Vernon *et al.*, 2004; Blumenthal *et al.*, 2005; De Jong and Gamel, 2006; Spanier, *et al.*, 2003; Denesh *et al.*, 2006; Kaushik *et al.*, 2006) and mental illnesses (Ost and Breitholtz, 2000) and acute stress disorders (Bryant *et al.*, 1999; Hembree and Foa, 2000; Sijbrandij *et al.*, 2007; Jain *et al.*, 2007). Brief relaxation regimes and mindfulness meditation reduces distress and improves positive mood states (Jain *et al.*, 2007). It is also suggested that a more relaxed lifestyle achieved through anxiety control can act as part of an overall lifestyle management scheme; this not only ameliorates the effects of coronary heart disease (Daubenmeir *et al.*, 2007) but also plays an important part in addressing mental health problems at primary care level (Greenstone, 2007).

Lifestyle management and brief relaxation

Coping with everyday stress surely requires an everyday coping strategy; however, often stress management programmes can be costly and are often used within secondary care settings within the NHS. However, only one in five with anxiety as a principal problem, ever seek medical help (Issakidis and Andrews, 2002). To capitalise on the unique adult access, the focus for stress control is now being directed at health promotion or prevention programmes delivered within primary care settings (Hickie and Groom, 2002; Roy-Byrne *et al.*, 2005; Greenstone, 2007).

Where relaxation techniques have been adapted to fit in with everyday life, there is increased compliance and use as compared to more complex or lengthy strategies (Krampen and von Eye, 2006). Further, having a technique that can be successfully applied '*in situ*' can reinforce a sense of empowerment or 'self-efficacy' (Hadhazy *et al.*, 2000). In the recent HSE (2007) recommendations, the workplace is increasingly seen as the setting by which many receive effective stress management (Eriksen *et al.*, 2002; Mackenzie *et al.*, 2006). However, there remain many adults who cannot access fundamental advice that bring the benefits linked to using simple stress management strategies. It is also evident, and arguably common sense, that techniques that are quick to learn and relatively easy to apply to general lifestyle will be the most likely to achieve the greatest adherence and therefore be of greatest relevance. The relaxation methods that have stayed the distance, in terms of ease of teaching, application and compliance, are those that are most portable to the setting in which anxiety is encountered.

Brief relaxation regimes cannot be considered a superior modality to ameliorate significant anxiety disorders; these are likely to require more in-depth strategies that challenge anxiety traits and negative cognitive attributes. This will require a more comprehensive cognitive behavioural approach delivered by trained therapists. However, there is mileage in providing a simple technique even while waiting for secondary NHS care. Stress control can be enacted as a prevention strategy for physical and mental ill-health, rather than, 'treatment'. However, this may create problems for maintaining commitment and compliance, especially in support of lengthy programmes. However, if the health care professionals have knowledge of straightforward techniques, there will be many opportunities to pass on some useful techniques for current and long-term use.

Portable techniques of relaxation

It has been argued that as stress management *per se* is a collection of strategies and techniques under a general educative cognitive behavioural approach, it is difficult to identify the most effective individual component (Marks, 2002). Most relaxation methods originate from progressive muscular (Jacobson, 1938), autogenic (Shultz and Luthe, 1959) or meditative strategies (Wallace and Benson, 1972). Individual techniques that regularly reduce blood pressure have best effects; importantly, this reduction can still be achieved through practising easily taught techniques such as using mantras or abdominal breathing (Parati *et al.*, 2002; Bormann *et al.*, 2005). Providing relaxation tapes even when well received by patients is not superior to being provided with a soothing music tape (Lewin, *et al.*, 2002). Indeed where a technique is passive, for example listening to a tape or receiving massage, there is some evidence that where there are positive effects, they are only short-term improvements, if at all (Hasson *et al.*, 2004). Jorm *et al.* (2004) reviewed a range of alternative treatment approaches, concluding that relaxation was useful in helping overcome anxiety problems with no one method or technique standing above others for effectiveness.

Education, education, education

The recipe for promoting active participation and compliance in therapeutic techniques is to understand *what* the intervention is, *why* it is effective, *how* to do it, and *when*. By promoting an understanding of the physiology and psychology of stress, an individual can have a rational as to why adopting certain behaviours can benefit body and mind.

The fight or flight reaction is often used to explain the reason why stress is part of daily lives, and it is often the bed rock of any stress management programme. A large number of web resources describes this basic stress reaction (e.g. www.thebodysoulconnection.com) which means there is little need to provide this information here. What may be helpful, is to describe to the individual how relaxation reduces the physiological effects of stress, leading to improved health and well-being (e.g. the lowering of blood pressure). This approach can motivate compliance with relaxation methods. Explaining the evidence supporting the impact of the different techniques, can also emphasise the benefits of a relaxed lifestyle. There are some excellent books that are suitable for client use, for example,

- *Managing Stress: Principles and Strategies for Health and Wellbeing*, by Brian Luke Seaward, 5th ed. Sudbury, MA, Jones and Bartlett Publishers (2006).
- *Stress Management for Dummies*, by Allen Elkin. Foster City, CA, IDG Books World Wide (1999).

The techniques that follow, are evidence based and suitable for use in a variety of settings, which makes them practical and suitable for most people. Further, they require no special physical capabilities, and do not rely on an external factor such as a recorded tape or complicated instructions. It is down to the individual to apply them when and where they wish. However, although relaxation exercises are useful, they are best integrated into recommendations to create and sustain a relaxed lifestyle. Applying all the available techniques cannot compensate for relentlessly living life in the fast lane, mistakes arise, tempers flare and self-maintenance is neglected. Lifestyle and relaxation must be synonymous, and therefore integrating the techniques into every-day life would be one way to achieve the more relaxed approach to life.

'Portable' techniques

Technique 1: Abdominal breathing technique (Advice box 7.1). This is the most portable relaxation technique. Breathing techniques can be performed by anyone and therefore must be the most frequently used technique. Yoga techniques and in particular 'Yogic' breathing has been used to reduce tension and stress for centuries, it has been found to enhance well-being, mood and stress tolerance (Brown and Gerbarg, 2005). Slow-paced breathing causes heart rate modulation leading to reduction in blood pressure due to reduced sympathetic and increased parasympathetic activity (Parati *et al.*, 2002). A high sympathetic tone in particular, is responsible for many physiologic abnormalities that collectively cause high blood pressure (Brook and Julius, 2000). There have been some studies exploring this technique in isolation of others with good effect in cases of gastroenterology disorders (Denesh *et al.*, 2006), hypertension (Kaushik *et al.*, 2006), lowering heart rate (Vernon *et al.*, 2004), functional breathing problems associated with asthma (Thomas *et al.*, 2003) and hyperventilation (DeGuire *et al.*, 1996).

The breathing techniques, in particular, lend themselves to be taught within an office setting, and the fact that a breathing technique is simple to teach and applicable in so many settings, has lent itself to being evaluated with a number of conditions. However, there is still the outstanding issue that there are only a few studies that measure its efficacy in isolation, and there is little evidence of how many sessions it can take, in order to master the technique.

Concentrative meditation

Technique 2: Tranquillity technique (Advice box 7.2 accompanies Handout 7.2). This strategy is derived from concentrative meditation techniques, which have been around for centuries (Perez-De-Albeniz and Holmes, 2000) a useful description is provided: 'Concentrative meditation techniques involve focusing on specific mental or sensory activity: a repeated sound, an imagined image, or specific body sensations such as the breath' (Cahn and Polich, 2006, p. 180).

Meditation that used to be based in spiritualism is applied more frequently today as a strategy to enhance well-being, with short-term benefits of calm self-control, and what Wallace and Benson (1972) called 'the relaxation response'. There have been reported physiologic and biological changes that take place, these include 'a wakeful hypometabolic physiological state and a balance of the parasympathetic or trophotropic and sympathetic or ergotrophic functions' (Perez-De-Albeniz and Holmes, 2000, p. 52).

The most common technique is 'Mantra' repetition. It is an easily taught technique that can be adapted to most environments, it has been found to significantly reduce symptoms of stress and anxiety and improve quality of life and spiritual well-being (Bormann *et al.*, 2005). By using imagery or mantras, it is possible to distract the mind from intrusive thoughts and thereby counteract ruminatory and anxiety-provoking thoughts. It can also be used as a distraction from thoughts that are depressive, negative and unhelpful, which can help individuals cope with depressive symptomatology (Lam *et al.*, 2003).

Technique 3: Touch technique (Advice box 7.3). This technique is based around a concentrative strategy which is derived from self-hypnosis, but does not induce a 'trance-like state'. Self-hypnotic techniques are an effective and popular strategy for pain relief such as in childbirth (Cyna *et al.*, 2006), migraine (Hammond, 2007) and can be a useful adjunct in helping chronic substance abuse individuals with reported self-esteem, anger/impulsivity (Pekala *et al.*, 2004). The technique follows the usual pattern of concentrating on a specific element (such as a sound or spot) and focusing the mind, which blocks out all other information coming into the mind from the surroundings. This can be helpful in scenarios such as dental treatment, and so on, however, it is not as practical as using an adapted strategy which allows the person to be able to move if necessary or be able to practice while standing at a bus stop or at their desk at work.

The 'touch technique' involves concentrating on one sense, that is, touch. Whilst the mind is concentrating on one sense, the information coming into the others is diminished, for example, when engrossed in reading a good book, the person can become oblivious to general noise in the surroundings, but the environment can come quickly back into focus. In using touch, ideally touching something like the back of a watch (most people have one), the technique is portable and readily adaptable to many situations in life. By focusing on the sensation of stroking the back of the watch, or smooth pebble/stone, can be similar to that of soothing sensation of stroking a pet animal, or for a young child, stroking their blanket/soft toy. The soothing action and focus of the mind on the gentle smooth sensation can help to reduce tension, induce calmness and can allow someone to be able to enter situations where (like at the dentist) although there may be no pain, the sounds and the sensations can be disconcerting. It is worthwhile if the health professional attempts all the techniques themselves, and uses supervision to reflect on how the techniques have been applicable to their clients.

Conclusion

Relaxation is now a concept that most can relate to. Many know what a state of relaxation is, but can find it is a state that is hard to attain, particularly in busy daily (and quite ordinary!) daily life.

Relaxation techniques are, essentially, strategies that one employs to reach a more relaxed state of being. There is a large body of knowledge suggesting that stress symptoms have a direct influence on morbidity and even mortality. Most often, the most useful stress management techniques will be the most 'portable'- those that can be used readily and are adaptable to a range of situations where perceived demand is being faced. The health and social care professional, often will encounter people who are facing demanding situations, or who, as a result of their anxiety, are seeking help. The most effective time to apply the techniques is when the anxiety is not so overwhelming that complicated and costly interventions are required. The relaxation techniques explored and described in this chapter, have been those that can be taught within an office environment, they are adaptable and convenient, and as they are effective, they can be empowering. Even if as part of a whole package of complex cognitive behavioural therapy, the techniques will stand the test of time, as they have been doing for centuries.

References

Astin, J. A., Shapiro, S. L., Eisenberg, D. M. *et al.* (2003). Mind–body medicine: State of the science, implications for practice. *Journal of the American Board of Family Practice*, 16(2): 131–147.

Barnes, Vernon A., Davis, Harry C., Murzynowski, James B. and Treiber, Frank A. (2004). Impact of meditation on resting and ambulatory blood pressure and heart rate in youth. *Psychosomatic Medicine*, 66(6): 909–914.

Blumenthal, J. A., Sherwood, A., Babyak, M. A. *et al.* (2005). Effects of exercise and stress management training on markers of cardiovascular risk in patients with ischemic heart disease. A randomized controlled trial. *Journal of American Medical Association*, 293: 1626–1634.

Bormann, J. E., Smith, T. L., Becker, S. *et al.* (2005). Efficacy of frequent mantram repetition on stress, quality of life, and spiritual well-being in veterans: A pilot study. *Journal of Holistic Nursing*, 23(4): 395–414.

Brook, R. D. and Julius, S. (2000). Autonomic imbalance, hypertension, and cardiovascular risk. *American Journal of Hypertension*, 13: 112S–122S.

Brown, R. P. and Gerbarg, P. L. (2005). Sudarshan Kriya Yogic breathing in the treatment of stress, anxiety, and depression. Part II – clinical applications and guidelines. *Journal of Alternative and Complementary Medicine*, 11(4): 711–717.

Bryant, R. A., Sackville, T., Dang, S. T., Moulds, M. and Guthrie, R. (1999). Treating acute stress disorder: An evaluation of cognitive behavior therapy and supportive counseling techniques. *American Journal of Psychiatry*, 156(11): 1780–1786.

Budh, C. N., Kowalski, J. and Lundeberg, T. (2006). A comprehensive pain management programme comprising educational, cognitive and behavioural interventions for neuropathic pain following spinal cord injury. *Journal of Rehabilitation Medicine*, 38(3): 172–180.

Cahn, B. R. and Polich, J. (2006). Meditation states and traits: EEG, ERP, and neuroimaging studies. *Psychological Bulletin*, 132(2): 180–211.

Carlson, L. E., Speca, M., Patel, K. D. and Goodey, E. (2003). Mindfulness-based stress reduction in relation to quality of life, mood, symptoms of stress, and immune parameters in breast and prostate cancer outpatients. *Psychosomatic Medicine*, 65: 571–581.

Cyna, A. M., Andrew, M. I. and McAuliffe, G. L. (2006). Antenatal self-hypnosis for labour and childbirth: A pilot study. *Anaesthesia & Intensive Care*, 34(4): 464–469.

Daubenmier, J. J., Weidner, G., Sumner, M. D. *et al.* (2007). The contribution of changes in diet, exercise and stress management to changes in coronary risk in women and men in the multisite cardiac lifestyle intervention program. *Annals of Behavioural Medicine*, 33(1): 57–68.

De Jong, A. E. E. and Gamel, C. (2006). Use of a simple relaxation technique in burn care: Literature review. *Journal of Advanced Nursing*, 54(6): 710–721.

DeGuire, S., Gevirtz, R., Hawkinson, D. and Dixon, K. (1996). Breathing retraining: A three-year follow-up study of treatment for hyperventilation syndrome and associated functional cardiac symptoms. *Applied Psychophysiology and Biofeedback*, 21(2): 191–198.

Eriksen, H., Ihlebæk, C., Mikkelsen, A., Grønningsæter, H., Sandal, G. and Ursin, G. (2002). Improving subjective health at the worksite: A randomised controlled trial of stress management training, physical exercise and an integrated health programme. *Occupational Medicine*, 52: 383–391.

Ewer-Smith, C. and Patterson, S. (2002). The use of an occupational therapy programme within a palliative care setting. *European Journal of Palliative Care*, 9: 30–33.

Greenstone, C. L. (2007). Clinicians' corner: A lifestyle medicine approach to anxiety and depression in primary care. *American Journal of Lifestyle Medicine*, 1: 167–170. http://ajl.sagepub.com at Leeds Metropolitan University, retrieved on 31 January 2008.

Gyllensten, K. and Palmer S. (2005). Can coaching reduce workplace stress? *The Coaching Psychologist*, 1(1): 15–17.

Hadhazy, V. A., Ezzo, J., Creamer, P. and Berman, B. M. (2000). Mind–body therapies for the treatment of fibromyalgia. A systematic review. *Journal of Rheumatology*, 27(12): 2911–2918.

Hammond, D. C. (2007). Review of the efficacy of clinical hypnosis with headaches and migraines. *International Journal of Clinical and Experimental Hypnosis*, 55(2): 1–24.

Hasson, D., Arnetz, B., Jelveus, L. and Edelstam, B. (2004). A randomized clinical trial of the treatment effects of massage compared to relaxation tape recordings on diffuse long-term pain. *Psychotherapy and Psychosomatics*, 73: 17–24.

HSE (2007). *Statistics: Working Days Lost Stress Related and Psychological*. http://www.hse.gov.uk/statistics/causdis/stress/. Accessed 1 October 2007.

Hembree, E. A. and Foa, E. B. (2000). Posttraumatic stress disorder: Psychological factors and psychosocial interventions. *Journal of Clinical Psychiatry*, 61(7): 33–39.

Hickie, I. and Groom, G. (2002). Primary care-led mental health service reform: An outline of the better outcomes in mental health care initiative. *Australasian Psychiatry*, 10: 376–382.

Hindley, M. and Johnston, S. (1999). Stress management for breast cancer patients: Service development. *International Journal of Palliative Nursing*, 5: 135–141.

Issakidis, C. and Andrews, G. (2002). Service utilisation for anxiety in an Australian community sample. *Social Psychiatry and Psychiatric Epidemiology*, 37: 153–163.

Jacobs, G. D. and Friedman, R. (2004). EEG spectral analysis of relaxation techniques. *Applied Psychophysiology and Biofeedback*, 29(4): 245–254.

Jacobson, E. (1938). *Progressive Relaxation; a Physiological and Clinical Investigation of Muscular States and Their Significance in Psychology and Medical Practice*. Chicago, IL, University of Chicago Press.

Jain, S. S., Shapiro, L., Swanick Roesch, S. C., Mills, P. J., Iris Bell, I., Schwartz, G. E. (2007). A randomized controlled trial of mindfulness meditation versus relaxation training: Effects on distress, positive states of mind, rumination, and distraction. *Annals of Behavioral Medicine*, 33(1): 11–21.

Jorm, A. F., Christensen, H., Griffiths, K. M., Parslow, R. A., Rodgers, B. and Blewitt, K. A. (2004). Effectiveness of complementary and self help treatments for anxiety disorders. *Medical Journal of Australia*, 181(7): S29–S46.

Kaushik, R. M., Kaushik, R., Mahajan, S. K. and Rajesh, V. (2006). Effects of mental relaxation and slow breathing in essential hypertension. *Complementary Therapy in Medicine*, 14(2): 120–126.

Kessler, R. C., Andrade, L. H., Bijl, R. V., Offord, D. R., Demler, O. V. and Stein, D. J. (2002). The effects of co-morbidity on the onset and persistence of generalized anxiety disorder in the ICPE surveys. International Consortium in Psychiatric Epidemiology. *Psychological Medicine*, 32(7): 1213–1225.

Krampen, G. and von Eye, A. (2006). Treatment motives as predictors of acquisition and transfer of relaxation methods to everyday life. *Journal of Clinical Psychology*, 62(1): 83–96.

Lam, D., Schuck, N., Smith, N., Farmer, A. and Checkley, S. (2003). Response style, interpersonal difficulties and social functioning in major depressive disorder. *Journal of Affective Disorders*, 75: 279–283.

Lambert, R. A., Harvey, I. and Poland, F. (2007). A pragmatic, unblinded randomised controlled trial comparing an occupational therapy-led lifestyle approach and routine GP care for panic disorder treatment in primary care. *Journal of Affective Disorders*, 99(1–3): 63–71.

Layard, R. (2006). The case for psychological treatment centres. *British Medical Journal*, 7548: 1030–1032.

Lewin, R. J. P., Thompson, D. R. and Elton, R. A. (2002). Trial of the effects of an advice and relaxation tape given within the first 24 h of admission to hospital with acute myocardial infarction. *International Journal of Cardiology*, 82: 107–114.

Luebbert, K., Dahme, B. and Hasenbring, M. (2001). The effectiveness of relaxation training in reducing treatment-related symptoms and improving emotional adjustment in acute non-surgical cancer treatment: a meta-analytical review. *Psycho-Oncology*, 10(6): 490–502.

Marks, I. M. (2002). The maturing of therapy: Some brief psychotherapies help anxiety/depressive disorders but mechanisms of action are unclear. *British Journal of Psychiatry*, 180: 200–204.

Mackenzie, C., Poulin, P. and Seidman-Carlson, R. (2006). A brief mindfulness-based stress reduction intervention for nurses and nurse aides. *Applied Nursing Research*, 19(2): 105–109.

McCluskey, A. (2003). Occupational therapists report a low level of knowledge, skill and involvement in evidence-based practice. *Australian Occupational Therapy Journal*, 50: 3– 12.

McKenna K., Bennett S., Hoffmann T., McCluskey A., Strong J. and Tooth L. (2004) OTseeker: Facilitating evidence-based practice in occupational therapy. *Australian Occupational Therapy Journal*, 51: 102–105.

McNair, B. G., Highet, N. J., Hickie, I. B. and Davenport, T. A. (2002). Exploring the perspectives of people whose lives have been affected by depression. *Medical Journal of Australia*, 176(20): S69–S76.

Mino, Y., Babazono, A., Tsuda, T. and Yasuda, N. (2006). Can stress management at the workplace prevent depression? A randomized controlled trial. *Psychotherapy and Psychosomatics*, 75: 177.

NICE (2007). Anxiety: management of anxiety (panic disorder, with or without agoraphobia, and generalised anxiety disorder) in adults in primary, secondary and community care. NICE clinical guideline 22, London. http://www.nice.org.uk/nicemedia/pdf/CG022NICEguidelineamended.pdf.

Ost, L. G. and Breitholtz, E. (2000). Applied relaxation vs. cognitive therapy in the treatment of generalized anxiety disorder. *Behaviour Research & Therapy*, 38(8): 777–790.

Palmer, S., Cooper, C. and Thomas, K. (2004). A model of work stress to underpin the health & safety executive advice for tackling work-related stress and stress risk assessments. *Counselling at Work*, Winter: 2–5.

Parati, G., Glavina, F., Onagro, G. *et al.* (2002). Music-guided slow breathing: Acute effects on cardiovascular parameters and baroreflex sensitivity in normal subjects. *Journal of Hypertension*, 20: S174.

Pekala, R. J., Maurer, R., Kumar, V. K. *et al.* (2004). Self-hypnosis relapse prevention training with chronic drug/alcohol users: Effects on self-esteem, affect, and relapse. *American Journal of Clinical Hypnosis*, 46(4): 281–297.

Perez-De-Albeniz, A. and Holmes, J. (2000). Meditation: Concepts, effects and uses in therapy. *International Journal of Psychotherapy*, 5(1): 49–59.

Persson, E., Rivano-Fischer, M. and Eklund, M. (2004). Evaluation of changes in occupational performance among patients in a pain management program. *Journal of Rehabilitation Medicine*, 36: 85–91.

Roy-Byrne, P., Craske, M. G., Stein, M. B. *et al.* (2005). A randomized effectiveness trial of cognitive-behavioral therapy and medication for primary care panic disorder. *Archives of General Psychiatry*, 62: 290–298.

Schneider, R. H., Alexander, C. N., Staggers, F. *et al.* (2005). Long-term effects of stress reduction on mortality in persons ≥55 years of age with systemic hypertension. *The American Journal of Cardiology*, 95: 1060–1064.

Schultz, J. H. and Luthe, W. (1959). *Autogenic Training; a Psychophysiologic Approach in Psychotherapy.* New York, Grune & Stratton.

Segerstrom, S. C., Tsao, J. C., Alden, L. E. and Craske, M. G. (2000). Worry and rumination: Repetitive thought as a concomitant and predictor of negative mood. *Cognitive Therapy and Research*, 24: 671–688.

Shamini, J., Shapiro, S. L., Swanick, S. *et al.* (2007). A randomized controlled trial of mindfulness meditation versus relaxation training: effects on distress, positive states of mind, rumination, and distraction. *Annals of Behavioral Medicine*, 33: 11–12.

Sijbrandij, M., Olff, M., Reitsma, J. B., Carlier, I. V. E., de Vries, M. H., Gersons, B. P. R. (2007). Treatment of acute posttraumatic stress disorder with brief cognitive behavioral therapy: a randomized controlled trial. *American Journal of Psychiatry*, 164: 82–90.

Sobel, R. M. and Markov, D. (2005). The impact of anxiety and mood disorders on physical disease: the worried not-so-well. *Current Psychiatry Reports*, 7(3): 206–212.

Spanier, J. A., Howden, C. W. and Jones, M. P. (2003). A systematic review of alternative therapies in the irritable bowel syndrome. *Archives of Internal Medicine*, 163: 265–274.

Stein, M. B., Roy-Byrne, P. P., Craske, M. G. *et al.* C. D. (2005). Functional impact and health utility of anxiety disorders in primary care outpatients. *Medical Care*, 43(12): 1164–1170.

Stewart, D. E., Cheung, A. M., Duff, S. *et al.* (2001). Attributions of cause and recurrence in long-term breast cancer survivors. *Psycho-oncology*, 10: 179–183.

Thomas, M., McKinley, R. K., Freeman, E., Foy, C., Prodger, P. and Price, D. (2003). Breathing retraining for dysfunctional breathing in asthma: A randomised controlled trial. *Thorax*, 58: 110–115.

Van Dixhoorn, J. and White, A. (2005). Relaxation therapy for rehabilitation and prevention in ischaemic heart disease: A systematic review and meta-analysis. *European Journal of Cardiovascular Prevention & Rehabilitation*, 12(3): 193–202.

Vockins, H. (2004). Occupational therapy intervention with patients with breast cancer: A survey. *European Journal of Cancer Care*, 13(1): 45–52.

Wallace, R. K. and Benson, H. (1972). The physiology of meditation. *Scientific American*, 226(2): 84–90.

Yogendra, J., Yogendra, H. J, Ambardekar, S., Lele, R.D., Shetty, S., Dave, M., (2004). Beneficial effects of yoga lifestyle on reversibility of ischaemic heart disease: Caring Heart Project of International Board of Yoga. *Journal of the Association of Physicians of India*, 52: 283–289.

Websites

Royal College of Psychiatrists: www.rcpsych.ac.uk/mentalhealthinformation/therapies/cam2.aspx
International Stress Management Association: www.isma.org.uk/

Recommended books for health professionals

Heron, C. (2001). *The Relaxation Therapy Manual*. Milton Keynes, Speechmark Publishing Limited.
Rout, U. R. and Rout, J. K. (2002). *Stress Management for Primary Health Care Professionals*. Dordrecht, Kluwer/Plenum Publishers.
Payne, R. (2000). *Relaxation Techniques: A Practical Handbook for the Health Care Professional*. Edinburgh, Churchill Livingstone.

All of the following handouts and advice boxes can be found as individual pdfs on the website at www.blackwellpublishing.com/thew

Advice box 7.1 Abdominal breathing technique (accompanies Handout 7.1)

Abdominal breathing is best demonstrated whilst the client is seated. Explanation of how tension in the abdominal muscles restricts breathing capacity can be illustrated by asking the client to tighten the abdominal muscles and notice how it is influencing their breathing. Many individuals do not realise how tense their body has become, often it is the gut area of the body that tenses first and remains tense even when the arms and legs have relaxed (say, when watching TV, etc.) Ask the client to 'let go of their tummy muscles' and even push the muscles out if they are unable to 'let go' of the tension. Then ask the client to place one hand on their belly button, the other on their upper chest (see Figure 7.1). The aim here is for the client to feel when they 'allow' their stomach to rise with the 'in' breath, that is their lower hand should rise and fall with the 'out' breath. The upper hand indicates if their shoulders/upper chest if lifting, which is an indicator that they have not released the tension in their stomach area. Breathing in through the nose acts as a limiter on the breathing rate, breathing out through the mouth allows the whole breath to be breathed away, but also relaxes the jaw. Placement of the hands is not necessary after the technique has been mastered. Suggest the client uses this technique regularly, in a variety of places (e.g. at home, in the car, at

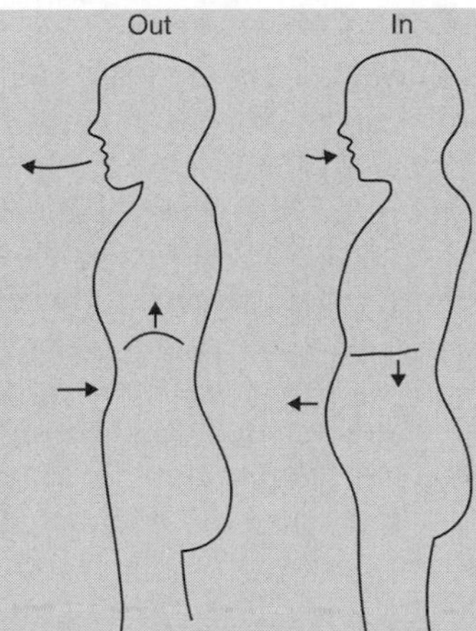

Fig. 7.1 Abdominal breathing technique.

the computer) even when not particularly anxious, this allows the technique to become more habit and routine than required coping strategy.

Often the client may experience the mouth watering, and/or a heavy sensation in the limbs, this indicates that blood is returning to digestion (hence salivation) and away from the fight or flight muscles (arms and legs). If dizziness is experienced, it is likely they are breathing too quickly, or breathing in and out through their mouth. If this happens, suggest that the client breathe out all the breath they possibly can, and then start the technique again.

Advice box 7.2 Tranquillity (see Handout 7.2)

The word 'tranquillity' works well as a mantra as it has such a strong correlation with relaxing, indeed, in looking it up in a Thesaurus, tranquillity is synonymous with 'composure', 'calmness' and 'serenity'. This word therefore associates with the state of relaxation. In addition, it is not a word that is frequently used in normal dialogue, and therefore can be used to associate with the imagery which you will introduce with this exercise. The other important note of worth is that words such as 'peace' or 'peaceful' can have an association with death or dying (as in 'Rest in Peace' which I found out to my cost in facilitating a relaxation group!).

Other words for mantras can be associated with the opposite, for example, saying 'relaxation' can be associated with 'tension'. This can undermine the goal of trying to use the word to focus on emptying the mind from thoughts which are stressful. In setting the scene for the client, it is helpful to explain that whilst this technique can be taken everywhere (i.e. portable), it may need in the first instance to be practiced with the eyes closed, until it can be mastered.

Advice box 7.2 Continued

Start by simply asking the person to think of the word 'tranquillity'; tell them to say the word in their mind three times, and then to associate a colour with the word. In my experience this is usually blue or green. After a few moments, suggest they think now of a place 'that means tranquillity to you'. If the client frowns, ask them to repeat the word until they can see some form of image – this can be imaginary or a real place that was tranquil. This technique then really moves into imagery – however, each persons 'place' is their own, this can prevent resistance in going to a place that might not be one of choice.

By asking the client to 'explore the place of tranquillity in your mind, using your senses' allows the mind to focus on a place of relaxation. This concentration removes the client from worrying thoughts as they will be unable to think of this image in their minds as well as the worry.

Advice box 7.3 One sense concentration: the touch technique

It is useful to advise the client that they will be using one sense to 'block out' the information coming in from the other senses (like reading a book) and therefore, it is not advisable to practice this technique when concentration is required (e.g. whilst driving). However, it is useful to accompany other activities such as travelling on a plane (when taking off and landing) as this can divert the mind from the surrounding noise.

Ask the client to find a smooth object that will fit in the hand. A watch is suitable, place the object so that the thumb can stroke the smooth surface, demonstrate this if it is not clear. Then ask the person to focus and concentrate on only one part of their body, that being the thumb, and the smooth object they can feel. Keep stroking the smooth object until the mind is totally absorbed by the sensation created by the stoking of the smooth object. This should only take 1 or 2 minutes.

If the client has remained quite still, and is clearly concentrating and not distracted, it will be clear that they are doing the technique effectively. Ask the client how they feel after a few minutes, suggest they practice this technique at home without detractions first, then increasingly often in a variety of settings, but not those that require concentration. Sometimes clients buy smooth stones/crystals which they find works even better, however, it might take a few practices to focus on this technique, and it can make some want to close their eyes, and feel drowsy – in which case, it can be used to induce sleep. Ideally, the client should only have one demonstration of this, and even if they do not manage to relax the first time, they should not use the therapist to totally relax them, this can result in the client only relaxing with the help of someone else, which defeats the object of being a 'portable technique' and undermines the self-efficacy.

Handout 7.1 Portable relaxation

Breathing to relax. Breathing slowly helps to slow the heart rate down, thereby reducing blood pressure.

Taking a breath in and out is influenced by the diaphragm. Hence, this technique can also be referred to as diaphragmatic breathing – it has been around for centuries and is often associated with yoga. Principally, it involves taking long deep breaths whilst the abdominal (tummy) muscles are RELAXED.

To demonstrate the influence of the abdominal muscles on the diaphragm, and therefore, breathing. You may want to try this exercise.

Pull your tummy muscles in as hard as possible; now take a breath in – notice something? You should immediately realise that if your tummy is tense, your ability to take a full breath in is impaired.

Abdominal breathing technique – instructions. You should be able to do this technique every where!

1. Start by breathing out through your mouth, as far as you can go, and concentrate on letting go of all the tension around your tummy.
2. Whilst your tummy is relaxed, take a slow, deep breath in through your nose – *this slows down your breathing rate, like breathing through two straws.*
3. Make sure that your tummy *rises with the in-breath* – this indicates that your diaphragm is falling down into the stomach area of the body. If the diaphragm cannot drop down far, breathing becomes shallow.
4. Hold the breath, momentarily, now breath out very slowly, through your mouth, let your shoulders relax, notice your tummy *fall with the out-breath – this indicates that your diaphragm is pushing all the air out of your lungs, allowing another deep breath to be taken.*
5. Try to do three breaths like this and notice if you feel heavier and calmer.
6. You can tell if you are doing this technique correctly, by placing one hand over your tummy button, you will notice your hand rising up with the in-breath and down with the out-breath.

Handout 7.2 Tranquillity technique

Distraction, using repetitive words, and imagery have all been found to help induce a state of relaxation in the body and mind. The philosophy is that when the mind is worrying, or dwelling on something that causes anxiety, the body, even if lying down or in a relaxing environment, will still react with anxiety symptoms. Therefore, if the mind is dwelling on positive, relaxing and worry-free thoughts, the body will follow suit, and let go of tension. This technique is essentially portable, you can take it every where with you! You do not need to be lying down in a darkened room, just be somewhere where you can spend 5 minutes 'switching off'. After practice you may well find that you do not need to close your eyes. The main issue is that if your mind is going round and round worrying about something, this technique should help break that cycle. As this technique requires concentration, it is not advisable to do this when doing a complex task.

The technique

1. Think of the word TRANQUILLITY.
2. Say it to yourself several times.
3. Think of a colour that you associate with the word TRANQUILLITY.
4. Think of a place that means TRANQUILLITY to you.
5. In your mind imagine that you are in this place of TRANQUILLITY.
6. Explore this place of TRANQUILLITY in your mind – what can you 'see' 'hear' and 'smell'?

If you have followed this technique, you mind will be focused on pleasant, warm and relaxing thoughts and images, and your body will be quite still, even your heart rate will have slowed.

8. *Lifestyle Factors in Managing Elevated Blood Pressure*

Jim McKenna

Introduction

This chapter will describe the contribution of different life behaviours and circumstances in altering and controlling blood pressure (BP) responses. The text will address which behavioural changes best modify BP difficulties without recourse to drugs. However, adherence to drug therapy is important to secure a reduction in worrying BP values. Typically, individuals are unaware of their problem although their behaviour can indicate problematic status even without diagnosis. Indeed, the behaviours that contribute to high blood pressure (HBP) are so common that they indicate how many people can benefit from changing their lifestyle.

Increasingly doctors recognise that elevated BP values may be a first signal that important other organs are under attack. A central notion for all to grasp is that once controlled, HBP is *not* cured, at best it is controlled. This underlines the need for continual vigilance in care and support. Reducing HBP, *aka* hypertension, is important not only because of the scale of the problem but also because drug therapy is so effective. However, drug therapy is expensive and BP values that do not justify pharmacological intervention can and should be managed through lifestyle options; the associated drug budget from Primary Care was £840 million in 2001, representing 15% of the primary care drug expenditure (Centre for Health Service Research, 2004). In the same year, HBP was noted directly or as a complication on 170,000 death certificates. More recently, a *Lancet* editorial (2007) reported that UK adults have a 90% chance of acquiring HBP during their lifetime, and in 2000 over 900 million adults worldwide had this problem (see Advice box 8.1).

Recently, non-adherence to drug therapy has been termed one of the unrecognised risk factors for uncontrolled lipid and BP problems (Lee *et al.*, 2006). In the UK, a wealth of studies highlight how most people with HBP go without medical treatment, emphasising the need for more attention to BP in adults (Centre for Health Service Research, 2004; Handout 8.1).

What is BP?

'Blood Pressure' describes the resistance of artery walls to blood circulating around the body. As cardiac output rises and arteries narrow, BP rises. BP is an important diagnostic index, especially of circulatory function. BP is altered by any condition or behaviour (such as smoking or exercising) that dilates or contracts the blood vessels or that affects their elasticity, or any disease of the heart that changes its ability to pump. Two nerve centres control BP, the cerebrospinal and sympathetic. Complex nervous mechanisms including pressure-sensitive structures in artery walls allow changes to local blood flow without disturbing general BP. The many mechanisms that influence BP highlight the wide range of lifestyle factors that might be adopted to reduce elevated values. This effect is important, since even individual BP measures are likely to differ from measures taken just minutes later.

BP is read at two points: the high point at which the heart contracts to empty its blood into the circulation, called systole; and the low point at which the heart relaxes to fill with blood returned by the circulation, called diastole. Pressure is measured in millimetres (mm) of mercury (Hg) using a sphygmomanometer, consisting of an inflatable rubber cuff connected to a pressure-detecting device; however, most doctors and nurses now use automated devices to make these readings. The systolic (SBP) and diastolic (DBP) values are given as a ratio expression of the highest value over the lowest, for example, 140/90, which, until recently indicated the threshold for 'hypertension'. When a single figure is given, it is usually the higher, or systolic, pressure because it is an important indicator of heart health, especially in men (Bowman *et al.*, 2006).

Normally, BP varies from about 80/45 in infants, to about 120/80 at age 30, to about 140/85 at age 40 and over. To support immediate survival needs, which typically involves meeting demands for energy (provided within the blood), BP varies between individuals and also intra-individually. It is generally higher in men than in women and children and is lowest at sleep (reducing by 10–15%).

UK population surveys suggest that hypertension affects at least one in three adults. In UK GP patients, 61% had systolic blood pressure (SBP) > 140 mmHg and in 77% it was greater than 130 mmHg. Of patients identified in the hypertensive range, 68% were receiving at least one antihypertensive drug (Williams *et al.*, 2004).

What problems does HBP cause?

Hypertension is considered a contributory cause of arteriosclerosis, which is characterised by a decline in the structure and functioning of the vascular system. Damage to the arteries associated with HBP can also result in hardening and thickening of the arteries (atherosclerosis), which can lead to a heart attack or other complications. Enlarged, bulging blood vessels (aneurysms) are also possible, leading to heart failure, blocked or ruptured blood vessels in the brain, kidneys or eyes. Poisons generated within the body cause extreme hypertension in various disorders, not least due to kidney problems. Abnormally low BP, or hypotension, is typically observed in infectious and wasting diseases, haemorrhage, and collapse. Systolic blood pressure (SBP) values below 80 are usually associated with shock.

Despite the range of pernicious associations, part of the difficulty in managing HBP is that it often exists without symptoms and has no known cause in up to nine in ten adults. For this reason it is referred to as a 'silent killer', although the negative side effects often do not necessarily link to premature death. Part of the reason for this metaphorical 'silence' is linked to the so-called rule of halves; only half of people with HBP know it (rule 1), only half of them are medicated (rule 2) and only half of them respond to their medications (rule 3) (Hooker *et al.*, 1999). Even allowing for errors in the scaling, the rule provides important avenues for skilful lifestyle intervention. Further to the problems underlined by the 'rule of halves' is is the problem of clinical inertia, which describes the lack of interest in effectively delivering treatments. Yet, epidemiological studies have confirmed that a 10 mmHg reduction in diastolic blood pressure (DBP) reduces risks for stroke by 56% and risks for cardiovascular disease by 37% (Centre for Health Service Research, 2004, p. 44). A recent summary of over 1 million men and women in prospective studies showed that for people aged 40–69 years every 20 unit increase in SBP (and a 10 unit increase in DBP) is linked to at least a twofold increase in deaths from stroke and other vascular causes (Neter *et al.*, 2003).

Prehypertension

A further development that underlines the need for more effective lifestyle interventions relates to a revision of what constitutes 'problematic' BP. With improved understanding of the relationship between BP and health, the ideal value is no longer considered to be 120/80 mmHg. The medical consensus now holds that any reading over 115/75 represents an increase in risk that is both progressive and continuous. In this new understanding of a graded relationship with a range of health indicators, the notion of 'prehypertension' is endorsed (Williams *et al.*, 2004). As values revert away from 140 mmHg the risk is also reduced (Julius *et al.*, 2006).

'White coat hypertension' (WCHT), which can influence up to one in three adults (O'Brien *et al.*, 2001), describes individuals who become hypertensive in the context of a medical consultation, but who are otherwise normotensive. This response is more harmful than might be imagined. A recent systematic review identified that WCHT patients had higher morbidity than non-WCHT patients, but reduced morbidity to that of established hypertensive patients (Khan *et al.*, 2007). This suggests that WCHT may be part of a continuum that ends with 'true' essential hypertension.

Special cases

Ethnicity. Given the responsiveness of BP to behaviours that change in different social circumstances, it is not surprising that ethnic groups demonstrate distinctive BP profiles. Internationally, ethnic disparities are known to exist in BP diagnosis, management and control (Hertz *et al.*, 2005). These profiles follow that of the general population, which rise with age and that are consistently higher in males. In the UK, higher SBP – but not DBP – values are found in the diaspora describing themselves as originating in the Black Caribbean (mean: males 133.3/74.7 mmHg, females 123.0/73.7 mmHg) and Ireland (males 131.5/73.9 mmHg; females 124.6/73.2 mmHg) (Sproston and Primatesta, 2003). In terms of hypertension prevalence, the national 2003 average was 31.7% of adults, whereas rates for the Black Caribbean adults were 38.4% and those for Irish adults were 36.4%. However, while national rates were lower in 2004, Black Caribbean rates remained above the national average (Sproston and Mindell, 2004). It remains unclear why these differences should exist, and bearing in mind that some ethnic groups consistently report lower average BP values, clues may be found in distinctive lifestyle patterns, differential responses to medical therapy or to adherence issues.

Male/Female. Women's Ischemia Syndrome Evaluation (WISE) (Marroquin *et al.*, 2004) has highlighted how traditional cardiovascular risk factors often play a stronger role in women than in men (http://clinicaltrials.gov/show/NCT00000554). For example, the so-called metabolic syndrome, which is a combination of increased BP, elevated blood glucose and triglycerides, has a greater impact on women than men, as does smoking, mental stress and depression. Finally, in pre-menopausal women, low levels of oestrogen represent a significant risk factor for developing microvascular disease also linked to HBP. These issues may link to a distinctive endothelial response in women.

Menopause represents an important transition for women, while post-menopause marks a stage when the coronary heart disease (CHD) prevalence quickly rises to match that of males. Compared with women who did not report hot flashes, those who did had significantly higher mean waking SBP (about 9 mmHg higher) and sleep SBP (about 10 mmHg higher) (Gerber *et al.*, 2007). Even allowing for effects attributable to age, race/ethnicity, body mass index (BMI), and menopausal status, hot flashes independently predicted average awake and sleep SBP.

Rising BP values are also problematic. Every 10 mmHg increase in SBP increased the relative risk of stroke among men by 19% and 15% for women, 17% for whites and 28% for African Americans (Brown *et al.*, 2007). Sexual well-being may be an important marker of an underlying problem and in men this is commonly evidenced by erectile problems. This alone may be sufficient to motivate lifestyle change in some men, but to avoid discussing it in others. Recent studies show that over half of men with HBP had some degree of erectile dysfunction (Albaugh and Lewis, 2005). Men with HBP may also have a low testosterone level, which plays a large role within sexual arousal. While HBP alone can lead to erectile dysfunction, some HBP medications (notably diuretics and beta-blockers) can also cause erectile problems. With the exception of avoiding activities prone to cause penile or groin pain, the key factors for reducing these problems through lifestyle are compatible with other recommendations for reducing risks of cardiovascular disease and BP.

Age. Recent Canadian data from the GENESIS study has shown that boys are more likely to develop elevated systolic values than girls (Dasgupta *et al.*, 2006). Cross-sectional surveys consistently show that BP rises by age cohorts. At the other end of the spectrum, HBP is not associated with mortality in post-85-year olds. That said, a history of high BP is still a risk factor for cardiovascular mortality in old age (Bemmel *et al.*, 2006).

Genetic jeopardy

Knowledge about the genetic effects of how well red blood cells transport sodium holds one of the keys to predicting the probability of hypertension, independent of gender, age and body weight. In the Rochester Family Heart Study (e.g. Fornage *et al.*, 1998) BP was more similar between people who share genes than those who did not, suggesting a strong genetic influence. This may highlight the value of family-based interventions.

Behavioural clustering

Research repeatedly shows that accumulating risk factors increases the likelihood of encountering disease outcomes. Further, the notion of clusters of behavioural risks is not only important, but also prevalent; only 15% of US adults were free of five common lifestyle factors – inactivity, smoking, low quality diet, overweight and excess alcohol consumption (Pronk *et al.*, 2004). Among 11,492 UK respondents, at least six in ten males and females reported two or more problematic lifestyles from smoking, heavy drinking, lack of fruit and vegetables in the diet and inactivity (Poortinga, 2007). Individually, lack of fruit and vegetables in the diet and inactivity were the most prominent factors. Each of these factors plays a role in regulating BP. Japanese data suggest that when three clinical states combine in the same individual – overweight/obesity, hypertension and hyperglycemia – average annual medical costs increased by 91% (Ohmori-Matsuda *et al.*, 2007).

Recent work (Siphai *et al.*, 2006) showed a continuous relationship between SBP and progression of coronary atherosclerosis. The closeness of these two risks for heart disease underlines the importance of lifestyle interventions, while also underlining the need to comply with medications. The Physicians Health Study showed that problematic (high) values of cholesterol (dyslipidaemia) are also predictive of subsequent BP problems in men (Halperin *et al.*, 2006). This supports previous work showing a similar position among women (Sesso *et al.*, 2005).

What are the lifestyle options?

It is important to understand the role of lifestyle change in reducing troublesome BP values and to understand that professionals' intervention can be effective. For example, despite concerns about clinical inertia, health professional's advice can be effective; when doctors advised hypertensive patients to change lifestyle, 59% subsequently controlled their hypertension (Primatesta *et al.*, 2001).

The Health Survey for England (Sproston and Primatesta, 2003) highlights a range of behavioural options. Among 5600 respondents, 806 (14.4%) patients had a 'higher than normal' BP reading the last time it was measured. Of these, 580 were being monitored by their General Practice staff, with 30.8% (175) already recommended by Practice staff to change their diet, 22.4% (n = 130) advised to lose weight, 14.5% to reduce stress and 8.4% to stop smoking. On the basis of these statistics it seems to makes sense to most health care professionals to promote the behavioural options that impinge on BP. Often the positive effects of such interventions become evident within weeks (Chiuve *et al.*, 2006; Roberts *et al.*, 2006). The worksheets in this chapter are designed to encourage behaviour change in clients based on the understanding that an improvement in self-awareness is the first stage in a sequence of events that lead ultimately to healthier, more permanent, behaviour change (Handout 8.2).

The lack of awareness of our individual BP is further complicated by the low appreciation of how valuable lifestyle change can be in helping to control already elevated BP values. BP elevation is mediated by adopting positive responses to high stress, poor diet and physical inactivity. These factors are each implicated in a distinctive cardiovascular response to different stimuli, whether their origin is behavioural, biological or cognitive. These same factors also underpin a variety of chronic conditions that support recurrent visits to health professionals. The relationship of HBP to diet, stress and stress-relieving behaviour is also profound. For example, stress can be linked to a disordered lifestyle – for example, inactivity, excess alcohol, poor diet and failure to comply with medical regimens – while the interplay of BP-lowering effects of these respective behaviours suggests the value of multiple behavioural options. Further, it is also important to note that much of what is known about how BP will change – and by how much – in response to specific interventions is based on strict doses and variable adherence. It is likely that the modest levels of change often reported from practice-based interventions (Centre for Health Services Research, 2004) are likely to be under-representations of the potential for more intense intervention. Indeed, even though lifestyle interventions typically only average changes of 3–4 mmHg, one in three adults achieve 10 mmHg change in BP through the same interventions (Advice box 8.2).

Regular monitoring

The only way to know individual BP is to measure it. This underlines the value of regular monitoring and shows that becoming aware of BP may be a first prompt for the need to change lifestyle. However, the invisibility and imperceptibility of HBP are part of the problem of acting to achieve behaviour change; with no obvious symptoms, there are no reminders of the need for continuous change. For this reason, monitoring can be seen as an important prompt for stimulating behaviour change. This can lead into careful planning of the first steps for making change. Part of this planning should involve how to manage the inevitable setbacks that accompany all efforts at change. Once change has occurred (whether or not BP is controlled) the motivational needs of clients will change (Taylor *et al.*, 2005; Handout 8.3).

Not only are individual office measures important, but the patterns of those measures are also important (Schwartz *et al.*, 2005). Many doctors now offer ambulatory monitoring which involves wearing a pack and an arm band, allowing; automatic recordings to be made throughout the day and night. Individuals who can access ambulatory monitoring may find it useful to explore variations in their daily BP and to locate what causes rises and falls in those measures. This will help to underscore the importance of lifestyle behaviours in regulating BP. To allow for any apprehension that home-based measurement of BP may create, values may be downward adjusted by 12/7 mmHg to equate to office measures made by trained professionals (Centre for Health Service Research, 2004; see Advice box 8.3).

Other BP responses take longer to show their effects and the length of the working day may be one such chronic factor. A recent large telephone survey found that extending hours at work to 51+ per week increased risks for developing HBP by 29% (Yang *et al.*, 2006). This response is graded compared to those who work 11–39 hours. Suggestions about why this may occur relate to how work impinges on other elements of recovery from work exertions and of adopting other more harmful behaviours, such as inactivity, increased alcohol intake and snacking. The ubiquity of government regulations about restricting work hours appear to have some implicit concern for employee welfare, even though many appear not to be enforced in meaningful ways. For health professionals, monitoring BP during work hours may be an important first step in supporting the other behaviours that also reduce BP.

Physical activity and exercise

Physical activity (PA) is used here as a generic term to summarise a range of behaviours, from formal exercise, to engagement in active behaviours (such as gardening or walking to work) and playing sport. PA in all its forms helps to influence many disease processes and body systems, including BP. Regular PA increases aerobic fitness although the behaviour (PA) needs to be distinguished from the outcome (fitness or 'exercise capacity'). Recent studies show how, even in the presence of hypertension (and high body mass index (BMI), high cholesterol and diabetes), risks for death are reduced in a graded response to increased fitness in both men (Myers *et al.*, 2002) and women (Gulati *et al.*, 2003). For this reason, the independent prognostic value of fitness testing (Mark and Lauer, 2003) may be justified within a comprehensive package of care for individuals. Even low levels of PA increase metabolic fitness, which produces beneficial adaptations to the many physiological and biochemical indices linked to CHD.

The Chief Medical Officer's Report recommends that all adults engage in at least 30 minutes per day of at least moderate intensity activity (like brisk walking) on at least 5 days per week (Department of Health, 2004) to improve metabolic fitness. It is of vital importance that all patients appreciate that their normal pace while walking in a park is often sufficient to create adaptations to our exercise capacity (Murtagh *et al.*, 2002). Despite this, recent evidence suggest that this message has not penetrated public consciousness (O'Donovan and Shave, in press). Importantly, regular exercise has recently been shown to increase levels of self-regulation, which lead to a range of further BP-beneficial behaviour changes, including improved emotional control, changed diet, reduced stress and alcohol intake (Oaten and Cheng, 2006).

A range of studies highlight a graded response of exercise on BP reduction (e.g. Iwasaki *et al.*, 2003). Accumulating PA is effective in reducing elevated BP (Padilla *et al.*, 2001) and, consistent with the need to promote a more acceptable 'lifestyle activity' message over 'fitness-based' activity, there is evidence that four 10-minute bouts of PA are more effective in reducing BP than one 40-minute block

(Park *et al.*, 2006). This is important since this pattern of activity can also lead to weight loss (Jakacic *et al.*, 1999), which in itself also improves BP control.

Active commuting is thought to increase total PA and epidemiological evidence for cycling for 1 hour (or for 25 miles) per week was associated with a 50% reduction in risk of dying from all causes over 10-years (Morris *et al.*, 1990). Further, cycling to work was associated with a 30% lower risk of mortality in both men and women (Vuori *et al.*, 1994; Andersen *et al.*, 2000). Benefits linked to cycling may be linked to its more intensive nature (compared to walking), which elicits a higher fitness effect. A recent meta-analysis of a more general effect of active commuting showed an 11% reduction in cardiovascular diseases, with stronger effects in women than men (Hamer and Chidi, 2008).

Recent evidence from the PREMIER study also supports lifestyle modification as a viable and effective option for reducing prehypertension. These data show the continued effects at 6 months (Svetkey *et al.*, 2003) and then again at 18 months (Writing Group of the PREMIER Collaborative Research Group, 2003; Elmer *et al.*, 2006). However, it is important to understand that prolonged hypertension may be associated with reduced capacity for exercise. For example, Shah *et al.* (2006) highlighted how declines in leg function were accelerated in 888 older adults (all clergy, mean age 75 years) over 7.8 years. Rates of decline averaged 30% per year for every year with SBP 160+ mmHg, compared to those with 120 mmHg values. DBP values exceeding 90 mmHg were associated with greater declines in gait. Collectively, these declines may be markers of HBP (or even mini-strokes) and can be used to signal the need to establish BP control.

Stress and job strain

Increases in job strain (characterised by the perception that work is dominated by high effort and low control) is often accompanied by weight gain, which is also associated with increased BP (Neter *et al.*, 2003). Risks associated with prolonged job strain were equivalent to the BP increases linked to inactivity in Canadian public sector white collar workers (Guimont *et al.*, 2006). While there are doubts that the specifics of the job strain construct may be the direct cause of HBP (Fauvel *et al.*, 2003), prospective data show that SBP reactivity was associated with hypertension over 20 years (Ming *et al.*, 2004).

Lack of sleep (Egan, 2006) is also linked to high BP, meaning that troublesome sleep patterns and allocation to shift working may all precipitate BP problems. In a prospective study of 816 employees, work-related stress in the form of a 'poor' psychosocial work environment doubled the risk of developing a sleep problem, while 53% of resolved the sleep problems were attributed to positive changes to perceptions of the work environment (Linton, 2004). Stewart (2007) identified lack of sleep as a possible factor triggering changes in the levels of intima-media thickness associated with subclinical atherosclerosis. While people may consider the impact of job strain on exercise behaviour, job strain had a more direct impact on healthy eating in 286 employees (Payne *et al.*, 2005). However, heightened job strain increased the consumption of 'high-density' snack foods, rather than influencing intakes of fruits and vegetables. Job demands affected exercise indirectly by lowering perceptions of behavioural control over exercise. Job strain was not related to exercise intentions or behaviour.

Interestingly, men seem more responsive, in BP terms, to job strain, making employed males a viable focus for coping-related interventions. Inter-employee behaviour and, therefore, workplace 'atmosphere' appears to be important avenues for mediating job strain effects. Local workplace group behaviour is another unexplored target for intervention. One Italian 'relaxation' intervention (Lucini *et al.*, 2007) achieved an average of 7 mmHg SBP reduction is employees in a company undergoing 10% redundancy, suggesting that health can be improved even in difficult employment circumstances.

Salt intake

International differences in rates of HBP are widely noted and many of these can be linked to salt intake, which is consistently higher in developed countries. In the UK and even allowing for differences between Scotland, Northern Ireland and Wales, while intakes are declining, they remain 50% above recommended levels, mainly due to a reliance on pre-prepared foods (Food Standards Agency, 2007). In some individuals, HBP is based on the responsiveness of the renin–angiotensin system, which is a hormonal system involved in kidney function and BP regulation. Up to one in four people with hypertension may have low renin angiotensin activity and for them the level of salt in the diet has a strong BP effect.

Diet/weight control

Diet is an important factor for reducing BP. Every 1 kg of weight loss is associated with 1 mmHg reduction in SBP (Neter *et al.*, 2003), underlining the value of regular weight monitoring and weight loss. Recent research has, however, questioned whether the link between obesity and overweight and HBP is as strong as previously thought; SBP increased by 0.71 mmHg less and DBP increased by 0.50 mmHg less in 2004 than in 1989 for each unit of BMI, despite large increases in rates for high BMI (Danon-Hersch *et al.*, 2007). This notwithstanding, there is a relationship between calories consumed (diet, including alcohol) and calories expended (activity behaviour). In untreated adults, each BMI increment of 1 kg/m^2 was associated with an elevation of 2.0/1.5 mmHg (SBP/DBP) in 1989 but only 1.3/1.0 in 2004.

In a range of recent randomised controlled trial studies, weight gain was suspended when exercise exceeded the equivalent of 10 miles/week of moderate intensity walking. Other studies suggest that a minimum exercise of around 40 min/day is needed on every day of the week, which is important given contemporary rises in obesity and associated diabetes. However, Kruger *et al.* (2005) showed that the positive role of PA is often underappreciated by individuals attempting to lose weight, suggesting the need for regular reinforcement during health care consultations.

In the DASH (dietary approaches to stop hypertension) diet (http://www.nhlbi.nih.gov/health/public/heart/hbp/dash) fruits, vegetables, and low-fat dairy products, as well as a reduced sodium intake are emphasised. Adults (n = 412) aged >22 years with SBP 120–159 mmHg and DBP 80–95 mmHg were randomly assigned to receive the DASH diet or a typical US (control) diet, consuming three different sodium intakes over 30 days each (Svetkey *et al.*, 2004). The DASH diet achieved BP control twice as effectively as controls (63% versus 32%). Throughout the trial, DASH conditions were more effective than the no-change controls. Comparing sodium effects within each dietary pattern, BP was 2.3 times better controlled by control individuals at the lower sodium intake than when they ate the control diet at the higher sodium intake. Maximum BP control rates were achieved in participants eating the DASH diet at the lower sodium level (84%), showing the value of a combined set of diet changes.

This study provides important evidence of the value of both the DASH diet and of low salt intakes. While, the study has limited application – because all food was provided to participants over 30 days of the trial – the average reductions in SBP (versus controls, mmHg) for DASH plus low sodium were –0.7, for DASH plus intermediate sodium –3.5 and –4.5 for DASH plus higher sodium. These findings are given further value since UK average sodium consumption is high (Food Standards Agency, 2007).

Recent prospective data gathered over 8.8 years in the National Health and Nutrition Examination Survey Epidemiologic Follow-up Study suggests that elderly men and women who regularly drink caffeinated beverages may be protected against death from heart disease (Greenberg *et al.*, 2007). This protective effect rose in a dose–response relationship where optimum protection arose from four or more serving/day (Uiterwaal *et al.*, 2007). These studies add to the growing evidence that caffeine, and particularly coffee may not be harmful to the heart, particularly in women and people with no other risk factors for the disease. However, these protective effects were found only in participants who did not have severe hypertension (i.e. not in those with stage 2 hypertension – 160+/110+ mmHg). No significant protective effect was found in participants younger than 65 years or in cerebrovascular disease mortality for those 65 years or older. In the Nurses Health Study I and II the caffeine in cola drinks, but not in coffee, was linked to hypertension in women (Winklemayer *et al.*, 2005).

Coping and relaxation

'Masked hypertension' describes the exaggerated BP responses to given circumstances (Pickering *et al.*, 2004). This, combined with white coat hypertension, highlights that individuals' immediate BP response to life events can be problematic. There is considerable evidence that the so-called mind–body relationship justifies psychological interventions based on changing how individuals respond to given events and/or how they resolve problematic responses to those same events. One in three adults achieve BP reductions of 10 mmHg by using relaxation exercises and meditation and there is considerable potential in using these approaches and in teaching them to clients who show an interest in them. These approaches may span from simply listening quietly to music (Chafin *et al.*, 2004), breathing more deeply, or even just closing one's eyes for 5–10 seconds.

Alcohol

Alcohol consumption is positively associated with BP increases. Patterns of alcohol consumption are also important, where consistent regular drinking is a more important determinant of the alcohol–BP relationship than intake in the previous 24 hours. A single intake of alcohol has a depressor effect on BP lasting for several hours, whereas repeated intakes for 7 days have both depressor and pressor effects according to the time intervals since the last drink. BP responses to alcohol may also be changed when drinking is the sole behaviour, or whether it is concurrent to eating a meal or simply consuming high-fat, high-salt snacks. Patterns of binge-drinking in the UK may mean that BP values are higher on Mondays than on other week days (Marques-Vidal *et al.*, 2001), which may help to determine when monitoring services are offered. Irrespective of timing, recommending low intake of alcohol is justified as a lifestyle intervention to reduce BP.

Smoking

Smoking is not a major contributor to BP problems. However, as part of a comprehensive lifestyle intervention, it offers important further health benefits, both for the individual and for people in their company. Giving up smoking reduces artery stiffness with attendant benefits for better BP Control. However, these effects take years to emerge (Jatoi *et al.*, 2007), meaning that prevention of initiating smoking is a priority (see Advice box 8.4).

Clusters of problem behaviours

Just as lifestyle clustering can increase risks for disease, behaviours can be grouped to amplify their beneficial BP effects. Important recent evidence, provided by the 18-month PREMIER study (Elmer *et al.*, 2006), emphasises that the multiple lifestyle changes (DASH diet, behavioural counselling and PA) made by 6 months can be supported at least to 18 months. This was compared to changes made by controls who received advice only. The trial was based on 810 middle-aged, sedentary and mostly overweight adults with prehypertension (120–139/80–90 mmHg) or stage 1 hypertension (140–159/90–95 mmHg). One important finding was that, beyond beneficial changes in BP status, concurrent behaviour changes were possible. A final further important point arising from this study was that 'advice only' was also associated with reductions in the numbers of people remaining in hypertensive states; the difference was just not as great as that produced by participants' further behaviour changes. This finding offers hope for all the lifestyle advice we might offer; give it because some clients will respond to it, even when we think our counselling skills might be underdeveloped.

Conclusion

This chapter has outlined the case for lifestyle interventions to reduce problematic and preproblematic BP values. A wide range of mechanisms are possible and the evidence not only justifies adopting interventions based on changes to individual, but also to multiple behaviours. These behaviours include PA, dietary change, salt and alcohol reduction and relaxation/coping, and each of these has a part to play in reducing risks for ill-health attributable to coronary heart disease as well as to those problems linked directly to HBP.

References

Albaugh, J. and Lewis, J. H. (2005). *Understanding Erectile Dysfunction: Patient Evaluation and Treatment Options*. Pitman, NJ, Society of Urologic Nurses and Associates.

Andersen, L. B., Schnohr, P., Schroll, M. and Hein, H. O. (2000). All-cause mortality associated with physical activity during leisure-time, work, sports, and cycling to work. *Archives of Internal Medicine*, 160: 1621–1628.

Bemmel, T., Gussekloo, J., Westendorp, R. G. and Blauw, G. J. (2006). In a population-based prospective study, no association between high blood pressure and mortality after age 85 years. *Journal of Hypertension*, 24: 287–292.

Bowman, T. S., Sesso, H. D. and Gaziano, J. M. (2006). Effect of age on blood pressure parameters and risk of cardiovascular death in men. *American Journal of Hypertension*, 19: 47–52.

Brown, D. W., Giles, W. H. and Greenlund, K. J. (2007). Blood pressure parameters and risk of fatal stroke, NHANES II mortality study. *American Journal of Hypertension*, 20: 338–341.

Centre for Health Service Research (2004). *Essential Hypertension: Managing Adult Patients in Primary Care*. Newcastle, University of Newcastle upon Tyne.

Chafin, S., Roy, M., Gerin, W. and Christenfeld, N. (2004). Music can facilitate blood pressure recovery from stress. *British Journal of Health Psychology*, 9: 393–403.

Chiuve, S., McCullough, M. L., Sacks, F. M. and Rimm, E. B. (2006). Healthy lifestyle factors in the primary prevention of coronary heart disease among men: benefits among users and nonusers of lipid-lowering and antihypertensive medications. *Circulation*, 114: 160–167.

Danon-Hersch, N., Chiolero, A., Shamlaye, C., Paccaud, F. and Bovet, P. (2007). Decreasing association between body mass index and blood pressure over time. *Epidemiology*, 18: 493–500.

Dasgupta, K., O'Loughlin, J. and Chen, S. (2006). Emergence of sex differences in prevalence of high systolic blood pressure: analysis of a longitudinal adolescent cohort. *Circulation*, 114: 2663–2670.

Department of Health (2004). *At Least Five a Week. Evidence on the Impact of Physical Activity and its Relationship to Health. A Report from the Chief Medical Officer.* London, Department of Health.

Egan, B. M. (2006). Sleep and hypertension. Burning the candle at both ends really is hazardous to your health. *Hypertension*, 47: 816–817.

Elmer, P. J., Obarzanek, E., Vollmer, W. M. *et al.* (2006). Effects of comprehensive lifestyle modification on diet, weight physical fitness and blood pressure control: 18-month results of a randomized trail. *Annals of Internal Medicine*, 144: 485–495.

Fauvel, J. P., Ignasse, M., Quelin, P. *et al.* (2003). Neither job stress nor individual cardiovascular reactivity to stress is related to higher blood pressure at work. *Hypertension*, 42: 1112–1116.

Food Standards Agency (2007). An assessment of dietary sodium levels among adults (aged 19–64) in the general population, based on analysis of dietary sodium in 24-hour urine samples. www.foodstandards.gov.uk/multimedia/pdfs/englandsodiumreport.pdf. Accessed 22 March 2007.

Fornage, M., Amos, C. I., Kardia, S. *et al.* (1998). Variation in the region of the angiotensin-converting enzyme gene influences interindividual differences in blood pressure levels in young white males. *Circulation*, 97: 1773–1779.

Gerber, L. M., Sievert, L. L., Warren, K. B. A., Pickering, T. and Schwartz, J. E. (2007). Hot flashes are associated with increased ambulatory systolic blood pressure. *Menopause*, 14: 308–315.

Greenberg, J. A., Dunbar, C. C., Schnoll, R. *et al.* (2007). Caffeinated beverage intake and the risk of heart disease mortality in the elderly: a prospective analysis. *American Journal of Clinical Nutrition*, 85: 392–398.

Guimont, C., Brisson, C., Dagennais, G. R. *et al.* (2006). Effects of job strain on blood pressure: a prospective study of male and female white-collar workers. *American Journal of Public Health*, 96: 1436–1443.

Gulati, M., MS; Dilip, K., Pandey, D. K. *et al.* (2003). The St James women take heart project. *Circulation*, 108: 1554–1559.

Halperin, R. O., Sesso, H. D., Ma, J. *et al.* (2006). Dyslipidemia and the risk of incident hypertension in men. *Hypertension*, 47: 45–50.

Hamer, M. and Chidi, Y. (2008). Active commuting and cardiovascular risk; a meta analytic review. *Preventive Medicine*, 46: 9–13. DOI: 10.10/16/j.y.pmed.2007.03.006.

Hertz, R. P., Unger, A. N., Cornell, J. A. and Saunders, E. (2005). Racial disparities in hypertension prevalence, awareness and management. *Archives of Internal Medicine*, 165: 2098–2104.

Hooker, R. C., Cowapa, N., Newson, R. and Freeman, G. K. (1999). Better by half: hypertension in the elderly and the 'rule of halves': a primary care audit of the clinical computer record as a springboard to improving care. *Family Practice*, 16: 123–128.

Iwasaki, K., Zhang, R., Zuckerman, J. H. and Levine, B. D. (2003). Dose–response relationship of the cardiovascular adaptation to endurance training in healthy adults; how much training for what benefit? *Journal of Applied Physiology*, 95: 1575–1583.

Jakicic, J. M., Winters, C., Lang, W. and Wing, R. R. (1999). Effects of intermittent exercise and use of home exercise equipment on adherence, weight loss, and fitness in overweight women. *Journal of the American Medical Association*, 282: 1554–1560.

Jatoi, N. A., Jerrard-Dunne, P., Feely, J. and Mahmud, A. (2007). Impact of smoking and smoking cessation on arterial stiffness and aortic wave reflection in hypertension. *Hypertension*, 49: 1–2.

Julius, S., Nesbitt, S. D., Egan, B. M. *et al.* for the Trial of Preventing Hypertension (TROPHY) Study Investigators (2006). Feasibility of treating prehypertension with an angiotensin-receptor blocker. *New England Journal of Medicine*, 354: 1685–1697.

Khan, T. V., Khan, S. S. -F., Akhondi, A. and Khan, T. W. (2007). White coat hypertension: relevance to clinical and emergency medical services personnel. *Medscape General Medicine*, 9: 52. Available from www.medscape.com/viewarticle/552593

Kruger, J., Galuska, D. A., Serdula, M. K. and Kohl, H. W. (2005). Physical activity profiles of US adults trying to lose weight. *Medicine and Science in Exercise and Sports*, 37: 364–368.

Lee, J. K., Grace, K. A. and Taylor, A. J. (2006). Effect of a pharmacy care program on medication adherence and persistence, blood pressure, and low-density lipoprotein cholesterol. *Journal of the American Medical Association*, 296: 2563–2571.

Linton, S. J. (2004). Does work stress predict insomnia? A prospective study. *British Journal of Health Psychology*, 9: 127–136.

Lucini, D., Silvano Riva, S., Pizzinelli, P. and Pagani, M. (2007). Stress management at the worksite; reversal of symptoms profile and cardiovascular dysregulation. *Hypertension*, 49: 291–297.

Mark, D. B. and Lauer, M. S. (2003). Exercise capacity: the prognostic variable that doesn't get enough respect. *Circulation*, 108: 1534–1536.

Marques-Vidal, P., Arveiler, D., Evans, A., Amouyel, P., Ferrières, J. and Ducimetière, P. (2001). Different alcohol drinking and blood pressure relationships in France and Northern Ireland: The PRIME study. *Hypertension*, 38: 1361–1366.

Marroquin, O. C., Kip, K. E., Kelley, D. E. *et al.* (2004). Women's ischemia syndrome evaluation investigators. Metabolic syndrome modifies the cardiovascular risk associated with angiographic coronary artery disease in women: a report from the Women's Ischemia Syndrome Evaluation. *Circulation*, 17: 714–721.

Ming, E. E., Adler, G. K. and Kessler, R. C. (2004). Cardiovascular reactivity to work stress predicts subsequent onset of hypertension;

the air traffic controller change study. *Psychosomatic Medicine*, 66: 459–465.

Morris, J. N., Clayton, D. G., Everitt, M. G., Semmence, A. M. and Burgess, E. H. (1990). Exercise in leisure time: coronary attack and death rates. *British Heart Journal*, 63: 325–334.

Murtagh, E. M., Boreham, C. A. G. and Murphy, M. H. (2002). Speed and exercise intensity of recreational walkers. *Preventive Medicine*, 35: 397–400.

Myers, J., Prakesh, M., Froelicher, V. *et al.* (2002). Exercise capacity and mortality among men referred for exercise testing. *New England Journal of Medicine*, 346: 793–801.

Neter, J. E., Stam, B. E., Kok, F. J., Grobbee, D. E. and Geleijnse, J. M. (2003). Influence of weight reduction on blood pressure. A meta-analysis of randomised controlled trials. *Hypertension*, 42: 878–884.

Oaten, M. and Cheng, K. (2006). Longitudinal gains in self-regulation from regular physical exercise. *British Journal of Health Psychology*, 11: 717–733.

O'Brien, E., Beevers, G. and Lip, E. Y. H. (2001). ABC of blood pressure measurement, part III. *British Medical Journal*, 322: 1110–1114.

O'Donovan, G. and Shave, R. (2007). British adults' views on the health benefits of moderate and vigorous activity. *Preventive Medicine*, 45: 432–435. DOI:10.1016/j.ypmed.2007.07.026

Ohmori-Matsuda, K., Kuriyama, S., Hozawa, A. *et al.* (2007). The joint impact of cardiovascular risk factors upon medical costs. *Preventive Medicine*, 44: 349–355.

Padilla, J., Wallace, J. P. and Park, S. (2001). Accumulation of physical activity reduces blood pressure in pre- and hypertension. *Medicine and Science in Sports and Exercise*, 29: 65–70.

Park, S., Rink, L. D. and Wallace, J. P. (2006). Accumulation of physical activity leads to a greater blood pressure reduction than a single continuous session, in prehypertension. *Journal of Hypertension*, 24: 1761–1770.

Payne, N., Jones, F. and Harris, P. R. (2005). The impact of job strain on the predictive validity of the theory of planned behaviour: an investigation of exercise and healthy eating. *British Journal of Health Psychology*, 10: 115–131.

Pickering, T. G., Davidson, K., Gerin, W. and Schwartz, J. E. (2004). Masked hypertension. *Hypertension*, 40: 795–796.

Poortinga, W. (2007). The prevalence and clustering of four major lifestyle risk factors in an English adult population. *Preventive Medicine*, 44: 124–128.

Primatesta, P., Brookes, M. and Poulter, N. R. (2001). Improved hypertension management and control: results from the Health Survey for England 1998. *Hypertension*, 38: 827–832.

Pronk, N. P., Anderson, L. H., Crain, A. L. *et al.* (2004). Meeting recommendations for multiple healthy lifestyle factors: prevalence, clustering and predictors among adolescent, adult and senior health plan members. *American Journal of Preventive Medicine*, 27: 25–33.

Roberts, C. K., Ng, C., Hama, S., Eliseo, A. J. and Barnard, R. J. (2006). Effect of a short-term diet and exercise intervention on inflammatory/anti-inflammatory properties of HDL in overweight/obese men with cardiovascular risk factors. *Journal of Applied Physiology*, 101: 1727–1732.

Schwartz, G. L., Mosely, T. H., Knopman, D. S. *et al.* (2005). Nighttime blood pressure level and diurnal rhythm are associated with cognitive decline. *American Society of Nephrology 38th Annual Meeting*, 8–13 November, Philadelphia, PA, Abstract F-FC095.

Sesso, H. D., Buring, J. E., Chown, M. J., Ridker, P. M. and Gaziano, J. M. (2005). A prospective study of plasma lipid levels and hypertension in women. *Archives of Internal Medicine*, 165: 2420–2427.

Shah, R., Wilson, R. S., Bienias, J. L. *et al.* (2006). Blood pressure and lower limb function in older adults. *Journal of Gerontology: Medical Sciences*, 61: 839–843.

Sipahi, I., Tuzcu, E. M., Schoenhagen, P. *et al.* (2006). Effects of normal, prehypertensive, and hypertensive blood pressure levels on progression of coronary atherosclerosis. *Journal of the American College of Cardiology*, 48: 833–838.

Sproston, K. and Primatesta, P. (eds) (2003). *Health Survey for England 2003. Volume 1: Cardiovascular Disease*. London, The Stationary Office.

Sproston, K. and Mindell, J. (eds) (2004). *Health Survey for England 2004. Health of Ethnic Minorities – Full Report*. London, The Stationary Office.

Stewart, J. C. (2007). Negative emotions and 3-year progression of subclinical atherosclerosis. *Archives of General Psychiatry*, 64: 225–233.

Svetkey, L. P., Harsha, D. W., Vollmer, W. M. *et al.* (2003). PREMIER: a clinical trial of comprehensive lifestyle modification for blood pressure control: rationale, design and baseline characteristics. *Annals of Epidemiology*, 13: 462–471.

Svetkey, L. P., Simons-Morton, D. G., Proschan, M. A. *et al.* for the DASH-Sodium Collaborative Research Group. (2004). Effect of the dietary approaches to stop hypertension diet and reduced sodium intake on blood pressure control. *Journal of Clinical Hypertension*, 6: 373–381.

Taylor, S. D., Bagozzi, R. P. and Gaither, C. A. (2005). Decision making and effort in the self-regulation of hypertension: testing two competing theories. *British Journal of Health Psychology*, 10: 505–530.

The Lancet (2007). Hypertension: uncontrolled and conquering the world (editorial). *The Lancet*, 370: 539.

Uiterwaal, C. S. P. M., Verschuren, W. M. M., Bueno-de-Mesquita, H. B. *et al.* (2007). Coffee intake and incidence of hypertension. *American Journal of Clinical Nutrition*, 85: 718–723.

Vuori, I. M., Oja, P. and Paronen, O. (1994). Physically active commuting to work – testing its potential for exercise promotion. *Medicine and Science in Sports and Exercise*, 26: 844–850.

Williams, B., Poulter, N. R., Brown, M. J. *et al.* (2004). The BHS Guidelines Working Party guidelines for management of hypertension: report of the Fourth Working Party of the British Hypertension Society, 2004 – BHS IV. *Journal of Human Hypertension*, 18: 139–185.

Winklemayer, W. C., Stampfer, M. J., Willett, W. C. and Curhan, G. C. (2005). Habitual caffeine intake and risk of hypertension in women. *Journal of the American Medical Association*, 294: 2330–2335.

Writing Group of the PREMIER Collaborative Research Group (2003). Effects of comprehensive lifestyle modification on blood pressure control: main results of the PREMIER clinical trial. *Journal of the American Medical Association*, 289: 2083–2093.

Yang, H., Schnall, P. L., Jauregui, M., Su, T. -S. and Baker, D. (2006). Work hours and self-reported hypertension among working people in California. *Hypertension*, 48: 1–2.

All of the following handouts and advice boxes can be found as individual pdfs on the website at www.blackwellpublishing.com/thew

Advice box 8.1 Asking about medication

Adherence to medication is about the most effective approach to BP management. Asking about adherence to medication could be included in every consultation with patients who have a known history of elevated BP values.

Advice box 8.2 The DASH diet

Where patients are responsive, encouraging them to adopt the DASH diet is warranted. It will not only bring benefits for BP control but also for weight loss and potentially, better adherence to being physically active.

Advice box 8.3 Encourage clients to choose their own options for change

Rather than telling patients what to do, encourage them to choose from the different behaviour change options or to generate their own options. This builds on their sense of self-confidence and affords them the autonomy they need to make good decisions that they can live with. Once success has been achieved in one area or set of areas, boosts in confidence will encourage further attempts elsewhere.

Advice box 8.4 Link behaviour change options to personal goals and ambitions

When discussing the potential of lifestyle change for controlling blood pressure, link the outcomes to things that the individuals value highly in their lives. For example, continuing to exercise might be motivated by wanting to be a good dad or grandad. Link any behaviour change to these 'higher' goals. To make this work well, spend time listening to individuals describing what they value in daily life.

Handout 8.1 Quiz: Are you at risk for developing HBP?

1. Black people are more likely to develop high blood pressure than are Whites or Asians.	True	OR	False
2. For most people, checking blood pressure every 5 years is adequate.	True	OR	False
3. High blood pressure develops only in tense, stressed people.	True	OR	False
4. If you feel fine, your blood pressure must be OK.	True	OR	False
5. If your blood pressure is below 140/90 millimetres of mercury (mmHg), you are OK.	True	OR	False
6. If your blood pressure tends to be high in the doctor's office but fine when you check it at home, there is no need to be concerned.	True	OR	False
7. If your parents have/had high blood pressure, you are bound to get it, too.	True	OR	False
8. Not adding salt to your food limits your sodium intake enough to control your blood pressure.	True	OR	False
9. Only older people (over 60) should worry about high blood pressure.	True	OR	False
10. The specific cause of high blood pressure is usually unknown.	True	OR	False

['False' is the correct answer to each item, except 1 and 10.]

Handout 8.2 How to establish the client's personal preferences for change?

The empty circles are to allow clients to establish their own options for change. Start by having the client complete the opening sentence about the main reasons for wanting to reduce blood pressure.

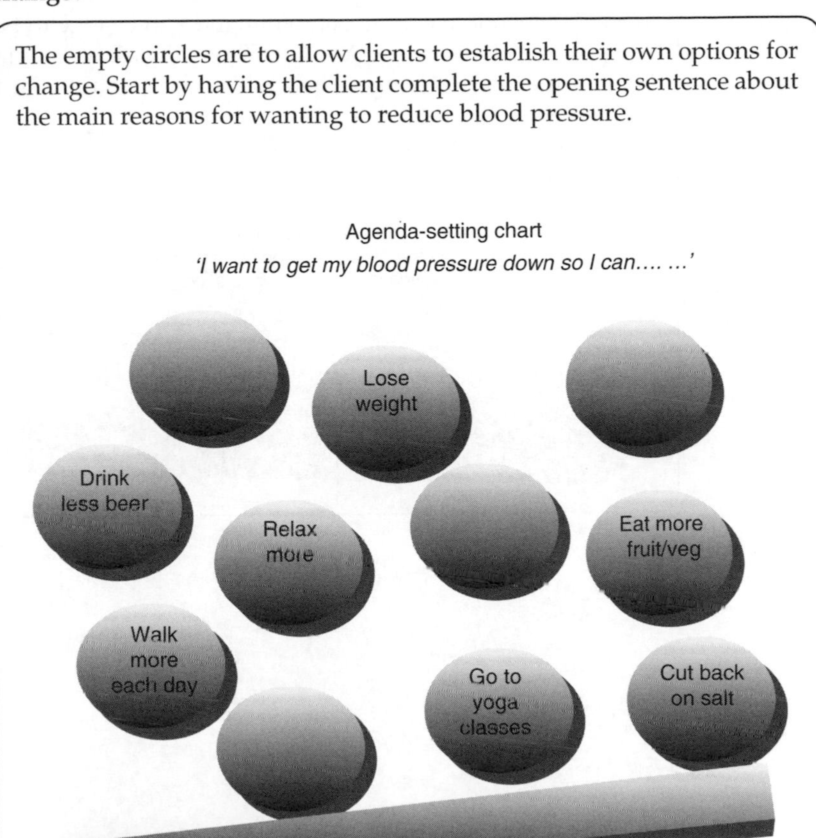

Handout 8.3 How ready is the client for making changes?

Once the agenda has been set, willingness to change to be developed using the readiness ruler. Ask the client to mark on the line where (s) he is in relation to change. Then ask what it would take to achieve a higher score.

Readiness (to change) Ruler

'I want to get my blood pressure down by... and my readiness for that change is...'

Not prepared to change

Already changing

Section C

HEALTHY LIFE AND HEALTHY RELATIONSHIPS

9. *Teenagers – Love and … Boundaries!*

Gill Coverdale

> The emotional atmosphere that exists between parents and children can lead either to constructive, healthy living or a life course fraught with missteps and obstacles.
>
> (Winnicott, cited in Korner, 2007)

Introduction

Adolescence is a very challenging time, both for teenagers themselves and also for those who are involved in their care and development. A parent's role involves more than loving and feeding their offspring, it also involves educating, nurturing, guiding, supporting and steering them through the trials and tribulations of childhood. Yet there is a lack of support and education to guide parents through this period. Understanding why children and young people behave as they do, and why they react to life's challenges in different ways, can help prepare parents/carers for a range of experiences they are often facing for the first time themselves.

The aim of this chapter is to explore the biological, psychosocial and cultural perspectives of adolescence in order to explain why it is such a challenging time. Contemporary government policy drivers will be discussed to explore how they are finely tuned to meeting children and young people's needs. It aims to provide a range of professionals from health, education and social care with information from policy and research which will help formulate advice and guidance that they may use with parents/carers who may be seeking help on an issue with their adolescent offspring. The information can also be used by the professional in proactive, preventative work, with parents/carers, or young people themselves with the help of the handouts at the end of the chapters (Handouts 9.1–9.3). Although this chapter does not explore the specific needs of children in the care of local authorities, it is hoped that the fundamental parenting issues raised here and identified by professionals early on, may go towards preventing that outcome. Where there is significant concern regarding parenting, there are a number of texts that may be relevant, for example, Hamer (2005) and Dunnett *et al*. (2006).

The bio, psycho, social and cultural perspective

Teenagers today

> The adolescent phase of the lifecycle refers to a complex terrain of intersecting biological, intra-psychic and social factors that contribute to significant transformations in an individual's development.
>
> (Hauser, cited in Taylor and Muller, 1995, p. 2)

This definition captures the complex enormity of growing up, yet despite all this, teenagers have a rough press. (The word teenager or adolescent is used interchangeably according to different writers but both indicate the teen years, 13–19). They are often subsumed into one mass and as the word 'teenager' can have a negative connotation, the whole of teenage society is condemned by the action of the few who are behaving in a disorderly and sometimes unacceptable fashion. It is undoubtedly an area in which there is a plethora of literature, yet it appears that society is struggling to manage this most changeable period of a young person's life. A recent international assessment of child well-being ranked the UK at the bottom of a list of 21 rich countries (UNICEF, 2007). The UNICEF report compared data in six dimensions: material well-being, health and safety, education, peer and family relationships, behaviours and risks, and young people's own subjective sense of well-being. When interviewed, England's first commissioner for children, Al Aynsley-Green said: 'We are turning out a generation of young people who are unhappy, unhealthy, engaging in risky behaviour, who have poor relationships with their family and their peers, who have low expectations and don't feel safe.' (BBC, 2007)

Parents and carers often ask for help and guidance in managing this challenging time of a child's life. This is well justified, there is an alarming increase in teenage alcohol, smoking and drug use (DH, 2004a; Social Exclusion Unit, 2004, 2007). There are also a high proportion of young people involved in crime and crime-related incidents, and the UK has a high percentage of suicides in the 16–25 years age group (Social Exclusion Unit, 2004, 2007; Young Minds, 2005). One tired father captures parents thoughts of the teenage years as 'a time of rapid ageing. Between the ages of thirteen and twenty, a parent ages twenty years!' (Pollard, 1998).

Biological growth

Atkinson and colleagues (1990, p. 100) suggest that adolescence 'refers to the period of transition from childhood to adulthood. Its age limits are not clearly specified, but it extends roughly from age 12 to the late teens, when physical growth is complete.' Adolescence is also seen to 'span the years between puberty, when the sexual characteristics begin to appear, and 18 the age of legal adulthood' (Fenwick and Smith, 1993, p. 15, in Turner and Helms, 1995). The biological changes are often the major indicators of the teenage years with the onset of puberty and all its facets. Girls in particular are now reaching relative adulthood before the end of their teens, largely due to advances in childhood nutrition and infection control (Bellis *et al.*, 2006). Other changes that occur are in the experiencing of pain, somatic and depressive symptoms, which positively correlates with age from 11 yrs to 17 yrs, and more so in girls than boys (LeResche *et al.*, 2005). In societal terms, however, the transition between childhood and adulthood appears to have accelerated in recent years, with many young teenage girls (and arguably younger girls) dressing in adult clothing styles, causing parental concern that their children are growing up far too quickly. Although there is considerable evidence that it is not the influence of media or fashion clothing but the interest that parents take in their teens that reduces the likelihood of children engaging in risky behaviours such as sex and drugs (Resnick *et al.*, 1997). Indeed, programmes that encourage parents to talk with their teenage children have positive outcomes in reducing the incidence of childhood pregnancy (Schuster *et al.*, 2006).

The social cultural and media impact

It has been argued that adolescence is a late 20th early 21st century concept, where we prolong child rearing and have our children dependent on parents long past the necessary age (Atkinson *et al.*, 1990; Giddens, 1990), whereas, only few decades previously, the child would have been expected to leave school at around 14 to engage in employment in order to bring income into the family. Perhaps, it is more that some of the difficulties of parenting occur as a result of teenagers having to 'unlearn' their childhood dependency and are learning to move from obedient to assertive. In our past, and perhaps in a more traditional society, the child would have been working alongside the parent, taking on more responsibility as they grew and aged, making it a much more fluid transition. It is argued that the world is a different place and children and young people now have much more freedom of choice and are empowered and encouraged to speak up for themselves. The cultural influences within Westernised societies such as the UK and US have been largely blamed for a negative impact on children and teenage well-being, with single parent families, being blamed for ill-health and disenchanted youth (Carlson and Corcoran, 2001). Indeed, the death of a parent is not considered as detrimental to a child as divorce in terms of becoming delinquent (Juby and Farrington, 2001). However, more recent studies suggest that teenagers brought up within a supportive community can ameliorate the effects (Kowaleski-Jones and Dunifon, 2006).

The way in which children interact in the home within their families is now dominated by media. What is becoming increasingly concerning is that children who are aged 12+ are occupying up to half their waking lives with some form of media (Strasburger and Wilson, 2002). One large survey in the US revealed that children aged over 7 years spent nearly all of their television watching time without their parents supervision (Woodard and Gridina, 2000). Although young people get a bad press in the media themselves (Strange, cited in Arnett 2007), it is increasingly evident that there is a direct link of the deleterious effects of mass media on children's health, behaviour and well-being (Strasburger, 2006a,b). The effects of media, particularly the Internet, on teenagers are only just emerging (Strasburger and Wilson, 2002). It is important that parents have technological skills to keep up with their children's knowledge, in order to ascertain the risks as well as being able to converse using technological and media language that children will be largely using. It appears, therefore, that what children gain in being removed from poverty appears to be at the detriment of time spent communicating within family units.

Psychological growth

There are many psychologists who have studied the psychological adolescent phase of growing up. Piaget was a renowned child psychologist who looked in depth at cognitive development, the way we develop our thought processes and make sense of the world (Turner and Helms, 1995). Piaget described stages of development: stages 1–3 address the cognitive development of 0–10-year olds; stage 4 looks at the formal operation stage, which is expected to develop between 11 and 14 years. Children in this stage are beginning to work out the consequences of their actions and conceive of possibilities beyond reality, they begin to solve problems by considering a variety of strategies and solutions and they begin to work with others to achieve. At this stage, children can be seen to become ideological and passionate about issues, such as vegetarianism, animal and human rights. Although it may seem difficult to believe for some parents, teenagers at this stage are very receptive to information that affects their future prospects such as money, jobs, friends and identity. This seems an ideal time to promote healthy lifestyle images.

Piaget argues that the stages occur in order and an individual has to move through one stage before the next can begin. However, he acknowledges that some people remain at stage 3 and never progress through stage 4 – they remain quite egocentric (selfish) and have concrete patterns of thought (everything is black and white). Arnett (2007) considers young people as 'emerging adults' who 'often have mixed feelings about reaching adulthood, not because they wish to remain childish but because they have discerned that becoming an adult has costs as well as benefits' (p. 28). Other psychologists have gone on to propose a fifth stage – a structural analytical stage – one of systematic reasoning and use of abstract thinking to create complex mental operations, certainly skills that will be required in the later stages of teenage years when at university or in vocational training (Turner and Helms, 1995).

Erikson (Turner and Helms, 1995) addresses adolescent development rather differently, although he still proposed a staged approach, each stage considers the particular conflict the individual is trying to resolve. Once again, one conflict having to be resolved before the next is attempted. As individuals journey through the conflict resolution process they gain characteristics, which help them resolve the next. Erikson asserts that adolescence is a time of identity versus role confusion; young people have to develop a personal ideology – an individual set of beliefs, values and principles that in turn provides them with a consistent coherent identity. But this battle, asserts Erikson, will rage as the average teenager develops their value system into a synchronous and uniform pattern. The identity crises and phases these young people go through are all a part of developing a role, which, at times is dependent on what is the 'in' concept. Arnett (2007) suggests that recently the view that young people spend their years in storm and stress has faded, but the identity and instability of their future causes some desire to assert their needs, and therefore, informing parents that all this is very normal can help divert crises in family relationships.

In learning who and what we are all about requires experimentation to see what the outcomes might be particularly in areas such as:

- Alcohol
- Clothes/fashion
- Sexual
- Smoking
- Drugs.

The nature versus nurture debate

Most young adults mature during this stage of development remarkably unscathed, but what makes those that do not different from the rest? One argument is the one of 'nature' versus 'nurture'. Research suggests that the environment has a significant influence on a child's well-being and the Acheson report (1998) proves that the link between poverty and social deprivation is stark. In the UK, 1:3 children are living in poverty. The physical impact of poverty is devastating, not only in terms of food and clothing but in the role of the parent and peers and the messages received from them (Wanless, 2003; Social Exclusion Unit, 2004, 2007; UNICEF, 2007).

Bee (1995) writes of the link between environment and heredity. If a child is born to parents with a relatively high intelligence quotient (IQ), not only is the child more likely to genetically inherit high IQ, but they will also inherit the associated wealth derived from it. In other words, where the child is more likely to have working professional parents, with a high likelihood of good housing, and a good school, they are likely to receive positive messages about what life can deliver. The converse of this is the child born to parents of a low IQ and the correlated problems associated with this.

School and peers are also seen to influence development. Peer-group can be responsible for the good or bad events in a child's life (Social Exclusion Unit, 2004, 2007). Children may throw away their family values and adopt inappropriate values which are detrimental to health and well-being. Teachers and school have a wonderful opportunity for exploration and information. The evidence suggests that children/young people are affected by the negative portrayal of teenage behaviour in the media, to the point of fulfilling the prophesy of the negative stereotype (Villani, 2001).

Facts and figures

In autumn 2004, there were around 5.5 million people aged between 16 and 24 in England. Of these:

- Around 750,000 were not in employment, education or training.
- Twenty per cent had a mental health issue, mostly anxiety and depression.
- Young men of this age group were most at risk of being a victim of violent crime. (Social Exclusion Unit, 2004)

Crime, truancy and exclusion

The Truancy and School Exclusion report (Social Exclusion Unit, 2004), notably Chapter 3, highlighted the fact that many truants and excluded pupils get drawn into crime with a three times higher risk of offending than non-truants. It also states that children commit 5% of all offences during school hours. There is a direct link between time lost from education and crime in later life, with a third of all prisoners having been regular truants from school and half of all male prisoners having been excluded from classes. Recent Government initiatives have looked at ways of reducing truancy in schools (DfES, 2006). Indeed, in November 2006, Schools Minister Jim Knight said:

> More than two-thirds of pupils with unauthorised absence miss five days or fewer.
>
> But it is disappointing that, at the other end of the scale, a stubborn minority of pupils remain determined to jeopardise their education and their futures by missing very significant amounts of their schooling.

(BBC, 2006 at http://news.bbc.co.uk/1/hi/education/5367240.stm)

The onus being on the joint efforts between local authorities, the school and contracts between pupil and parent, including punishment of the parent where the contract is breached (DfES, 2003). This may decrease the truancy statistics; however, there is little government investment in addressing the reasons behind such persistent truancy.

Teenage pregnancy

Willcox and Gleeson (2003) found that between a third and a half of all sexually active young people do not use contraception at first intercourse. This increases their chance of conceiving within a year to 90%. Children born to teenage mothers generally face disadvantages: they are more likely to die in infancy, have poor health and do badly at school; daughters of teenage mothers are more likely to become teenage mothers themselves, continuing the cycle of early parenthood and social exclusion (Teenage Pregnancy Unit, 2004; DfES, 2007).

Parenting is a highly demanding role requiring support from family and friends, emotional maturity to manage the challenging times ahead and financial security. The 'Teenage Pregnancy Report' (2004) claims that these key requirements are not always present in a teenage pregnancy and parenthood. Preventing unwanted pregnancies is a key government target and one that has clear frameworks for addressing the problem, building on the successes of projects around the UK (DH, 2007). Parents' influence through their attitudes and behaviours have a serious impact on teenagers sexual health. Children's sexual behaviour can be influenced positively by parents discussing sexuality topics with their children before they engage in romantic relationships (Eisenberg *et al.*, 2006); empowering parents to develop effective and positive relationships with their children can work towards addressing the problem (Every Child Matters, 2007). The government's ambition is that all young people should have the skills, confidence and motivation to look after their sexual health and delay parenthood until they are in a better position – emotionally, educationally and economically – to face its challenges. Reassuringly the target to reduce teenage pregnancies is slowly being reached, to the point where both the under-18 years and under-16 years conception rates are at their lowest levels for 20 years (see Box 9.1).

Box 9.1 Teenage conception statistics for England, 1998–2005

- The provisional 2005 under-18 conception rate for England of 41.1 per 1000 girls aged 15–17 represents an overall decline of 11.8% since 1998 – the baseline year for the Teenage Pregnancy Strategy.
- The provisional under 16 conception rate for England in 2005 was 7.8 per 1000 girls aged 13–15. This is 12.1% lower than the Teenage Pregnancy Strategy's 1998 baseline rate of 8.8 conceptions per 1000 girls aged 13–15.

Source: From the Teenage Pregnancy Unit (DH, 2007).

The government policy drivers

There is a plethora of policy documentation from health, education and social care agencies collaboratively advocating professional support to meet the needs of children, young people and their families (Acheson, 1998; DH, 2002, 2004a,b; DH, DfES, 2003a,b, 2005a,b,c; Wanless, 2003). Yet it is argued that under-investment in children means we still have twice the number of children living below the poverty line than in 1979 (Bradshaw, 2007). The following selection of policy documentation is recommended for professionals to gain a comprehensive understanding of the direction of children's services:

- Every Child Matters (DH, DfES 2003a)
- National Service Framework for Children and Young People (DH 2004b)
- Keeping Children Safe (DH, DfES 2003b)
- Youth Matters (DfES, 2005b)
- Healthy Living Blueprint (DfES, 2004a)
- Chief Nursing Officer review of vulnerable children and young people (DH, 2004c).

Education has the opportunity to make a major contribution to children and young people's life choices, confidence, self-awareness and ultimately to influence their self-esteem. The extended schools (DfES, 2005a) and healthy schools agenda (DfES, 2005b), generated as part of the 'Every Child Matters' policy drive (DH, DfES, 2003a), are promoting health and well-being, and ensuring that opportunities are provided for children to reach their full potential. Schools located at the heart of the community are well placed to take up the challenge of making Every Child Matters a reality for children, young people and communities, providing child care, before and after school activities for children and providing parents and other members of the community opportunities to learn and develop skills. Research has shown that schools providing extended services can expect improvements in performance (DH, DfES, 2003a). A thematic review (DfES, 2005c) of the evaluation of full service extended schools shows that extended services can have significant positive effects on children, adults and families. These effects can also benefit schools – improving pupil attainment, self-esteem and exclusion rates.

Key issues for children and young people

The key government policy issues for young people are sexual health and relationship education, mental health and well-being, and education and information on drugs, alcohol and substance misuse. These are all addressed through the Personal and Social Health Education programme at school (DfES, 2006). This does not mean education on these issues should not go beyond the school gates. It is my view that if parents talk with and build good relationships with their children it can be one of the biggest defences in the armoury of tools to combat disaffection and abuse. The government has recognised this and acknowledged that parents need support in this area and has set out a range of strategies in its policy document '*Support for Parents: The Best Start for Children*' (DH, 2006a), with the emphasis being on prevention rather than treatment in an effort to break the cycle of disadvantage.

Four key guiding principles will inform the government's approach and actions:

- Better identification and earlier intervention
- Systematically identifying 'what works'
- Promoting multi-agency working
- Personalisation, rights and responsibilities.

Source: DH (2006a,b).

Developing parenting skills

Parenting is a multiplex concept, with cultural and social contextualisation (Kendall and Blookfield, 2005) influencing the type of parenting and the success of parenting. There is little evidence of local authorities providing parenting classes *per se*, however, there are family therapy services for whole families of 'problem' children. Picking up the skills and knowledge on how to be a 'good enough parent' is extremely *ad hoc*. This suggests that there is little in the prevention of mental ill-health in teenagers.

There has been a growth of research into the use of parenting skills programmes and their value, with evidence that parenting programmes can contribute to improving children's behaviour. Parenting programmes aim to empower and enable parents to utilise problem-solving approaches and understand their children's behaviour and how their own behaviour impacts on this. Long *et al.* (2001) research showed that after an 8-week parenting skills programme, participants revealed that they found they had reduced levels of anxiety and depression, used less punitive sanctions such as shouting, felt an improvement in the calm atmosphere in the home environment and an increase in the use of problem-focused coping strategies.

Improving communication with children, with strategies to deal with difficult behaviour and developing responsible discipline using consequences, reported improved confidence and self-esteem in parents (Long *et al.*, 2001; Hallam *et al.*, 2006; Parker and Kirk, 2006).

Parker and Kirk (2006) describe the empowerment model of the Parent Positive Programme, which they developed to raise self-esteem and develop parenting skills through the use of a home-based Health Needs Assessment questionnaire. This was used by health visitors in the home, allowing parents and carers to examine and identify factors influencing family life and solutions to resolving problems. DELTA (Developing Everyone's Learning and Thinking Abilities) is a programme developed by Jones (2006) to promote holistic development of children's and parent's self-esteem, and improving relationships, through the 'parents as partners' model. This centres on communicating, listening and sharing learning opportunities such as reading and playing together, this would be easy to continue into adolescence.

Although Local Authorities can use its power to impose parenting orders to address poor behaviour (Anti-social Behaviour Act, 2003), these can involve enforced attendance at parenting classes which presents a negative slant. The use of behavioural and 'improving relationships' approaches have been seen to contribute to improving children's behaviour and 'at home good parenting', which can have significant positive effects on achievement (Hallam *et al.*, 2006).

A US-based child and parenting programme (Webster-Stratton and Hammond, 1997) advocates play, confidence building, healthy eating and lifestyle as key constructs in managing relationships which can build harmony into aggressive households. The 'Family Links Nurturing Programme' (Hunt and Mountford, 2003) suggests the use of praise, rules, building self-esteem and skills to problem solve, along with self-awareness, reasonable expectations, empathy and positive discipline. These are all effective and achievable strategies to enhance family relationships.

Gillies' (2006) research comparing working and middle-class parents offers insight into the role of social class and child rearing. It illustrates how promoting parenting skills without taking into account the normative, culturally specific assumptions about what constitutes good parenting obscures the social class differences. She argues that exploration into parenting reveals a different slant on the three key laments of poor parenting:

- Disinvestment in schooling
- Defending poor behaviour
- Provision of inappropriate treats.

She highlights notably different values between the two groups, for example, kindness and good behaviour being as highly ranked as 'smart' in the working-class group. She advises that parenting programmes be designed with social class in mind.

Parenting skills can be taught to teenagers at school. Stepping Stones (Harrison *et al.*, 2005) is a Bradford-based venture started by a School Nurse and Health Visitor with high-school pupils to improve parenting skills and prevent teenage pregnancies. It is now in the community in partnership with other health workers and local volunteer mums. Skill mix is seen as the key to success and the mums involved have agreed they have learnt a few tricks on parenting themselves.

Kendall and Blookfield (2005) evaluated the effectiveness of parenting programmes arguing a dearth of research in this field due to its outcome-focused approach and also a lack of rigour in research, such as small samples or overreliance of self-reporting. However, programmes providing parenting skills, relationship-building techniques, behaviour management training, in collaboration with children, families, schools and professionals from health and social care are likely to provide the strongest, most applicable and locally accessible programmes.

Improving and developing good communication

Adults listening actively with interest is of vital importance to children and young people and is an opportunity for parents/ carers to stay involved even if they are no longer involved in events or activities with their teenager. This obvious piece of advice needs to be encouraged and promoted in the current social climate of TV dinners and lack of formal dining space/time and long working week. Many families report that they are spending little time socialising together.

Communicating and consulting with children and young people seems the most logical way to approach difficulties between parents and young people, however, with the emotional upheavals of adolescence it is a difficult process. Korner (2007) suggests it is often the one important element that is overlooked or attempted unsuccessfully. He suggests this is because of the failure to master the art of listening without allowing the emotions to overrule the listening. Korner states:

> Parents and children reciprocally exchange or "catch" emotions from each other. Emotions are contagious and are often caught just like colds. Once parents and children "infect" each other with an emotion (i.e. frustration; anger; sadness), the job of emotional regulation becomes more complex.

He advises that these emotions are kept in check or are held at bay so that premature, punitive actions do not invade and disrupt (shouting, threatening) the communication. The way words are delivered can have more impact than what is actually said. Therefore, to prevent crises in family life, advise parents and young people to take some time out when communication is not going to plan and resume when everyone has calmed down.

Exploring together what the problems are can help to identify obstacles for moving forward. Children and young people often 'use' a behavioural pattern in lieu of expressing a feeling that is intolerable to them or their parents for example disrespect, swearing, underachievement or oppositional/defiant behaviour (Korner, 2007). As most children are protective of their parents even when their relationship appears to be very negative, they will benefit from expressing the feelings in words rather than action that have been deemed 'taboo'. If this is managed well (and it may need a third person to act as an intermediary) the behaviours become unnecessary and drop off by themselves (Korner, 2007).

Parenting advice and guidance

Reassuringly, for parents/carers and professionals, there is help at hand from varying sources. There has been an increase in, and development of, parenting groups, classes and one-to-one support services such as KidScope (a multi-agency service where parents and teachers can seek advice and guidance before problems escalate). School nurses are an excellent resource for schools, young people and their parents for addressing issues early and for providing support and advice strategies as well as for utilising their close links with Child and Adolescent Mental Health Services (CAMHS) and other agencies to refer to if problems escalate (DH, 2006b). General practitioners (GPs) and practice nurses are also key professionals available for advice and guidance and signposting on to other services if required; in school, learning mentors are providing a vital link between the young person, school and home.

The Royal College of Psychiatrists have produced a useful range of resources to guide professionals, young people and their parents. The fact-sheets provide guidance and tips for parenting and for young people in coping with their parents! The National Society for the Prevention of Cruelty to Children (NSPCC) and Parentline are also a major source of guidance. A summary of these resources are provided in Advice box 9.1, which readers can use with their clients. Guidance can also be sought from the National Institute for Clinical Excellence (NICE) and other publications especially where the issues are more complex: these are listed in Advice box 9.2.

Conclusion

Adolescence is a period of great change – physically, intellectually, emotionally and socially. It is a challenging time for families and as a society arguably a challenge we need to address. There is an alarming increase in the number of young people turning to crime and ineffective lifestyles. The UNICEF (2007) report reveals that many of the children and young people in the UK do not feel loved, cherished, supported or valued. Yet, recent studies (RCP, 2007) suggest teenagers turn to their parents most in times of need, and although these years can be difficult, the vast majority of teenagers grow up into happy, healthy, successful adults.

Society today is vastly changed from when most parents were children and teenagers, and the choices and decisions they need to make are more complex in some ways. As a society, we need to value these individuals and support them through these formative years if we are to reap the benefits of them as adults; it requires investment from all agencies. We need to understand teenagers and empathise with the challenges they face. In the last millennium, we have given children more power and more knowledge and skills than our forefathers; we have empowered them to have a voice, the world is a different place and of course they are going to react differently to it.

We have to understand and shape their need to push against the boundaries set; we need to be there for them when the experimenting is over. How do we do this effectively? Health and social care professionals work with parents and often teenagers in a range of contexts; with an understanding of young people's needs, we can promote adolescence as a positive time which provides parents with opportunities to shape their children's future, celebrate their achievements and improve their self-worth.

References

Acheson, D. (1998). *Independent Inquiry into Inequalities in Health.* Accessed September 2007: http://www.archive.official-documents.co.uk/document/doh/ih/ih.htm. London, HMSO.

Arnett, J. J. (2007). Suffering, selfish, slackers? Myths and reality about emerging adults. *Journal of Youth Adolescence*, 36: 23–29.

Atkinson, R. L., Atkinson, R. C., Smith, E. E., Benn, D. J. and Hilgard, E. R. (1990). *Introduction to Psychology*, 10th edition. Florida, Harcourt Brace.

BBC (2007). *BBC News: UK Accused of Failing Children.* Accessed from http://newsvote.bbc.co.uk/mpapps/pagetools/print/news.bbc.co.uk/1/hi/uk/6359363.stm on 14/2/2007.

Bee, H. (1995). *The Growing Child.* New York, Harper Collins.

Bellis, M. A., Downing, J. and Ashton, J. R. (2006). Adults at 12? Trends in puberty and their public health consequences. *Journal of Epidemiology and Community Health*, 60: 910–911.

Bradshaw, J. (2007) *BBC News: UK is Accused of Failing Children.* http://newsvote.bbc.co.uk/mpapps/pagetools/print/news.bbc.co.uk/1/hi/uk/6359363.stm

Carlson, M. J. and Corcoran, M. E. (2001). Family structure and children's behavioral and cognitive outcomes. *Journal of Marriage and the Family*, 63(3): 779–792.

DfEE (2001). *Promoting Children's Mental Health within Early Years and School Settings.* London, Department for Education and Employment.

DfES (2003). *Guidance on Education Related Parenting Contract, Parenting Orders and Penalty Notices.* London, Department for Education and Skills.

DfES (2004). *A Healthy Living Blueprint.* London, The Stationary Office.

DfES (2005a). *Extended Schools – Access to Opportunities and Services for All. A Prospectus.* London, Department for Education and Skills.

DfES (2005b). *Youth Matters – Green Paper.* London, The Stationary Office.

DfES (2005c). *National Healthy Schools Programme.* http://www.healthy-schools.gov.uk. London, Department for Education and Skills.

DfES (2006). *Support for Parents: The Best Chance for Children.* http://www.hm-treasury.gov.uk./media/5/E/pbr05_supportparents_391.pdf. London, Department for Education and Skills.

DfES (2007). *Teenage Parents Next Steps: Guidance for Local Authorities and Primary Care Trusts.* London, Department for Education and Skills.

DH (2002). *Action Plan: Core Principles for the Involvement of Children and Young People.* http://www.dh.gov.uk/en/Publicationsandstatistics/Publications/PublicationsPolicyAndGuidance/DH_4008816. London, Department of Health.

DH (2004a). *Choosing Health.* London, HMSO.

DH (2004b). *The National Service Framework for Children and Young People.* London, The Stationary Office.

DH (2004c). *Chief Nursing Officer Review of Vulnerable Children and Young People.* London, The Stationary Office.

DH (2006a). *Support for Parents: The Best Start for Children* at http://www.hm-treasury.gov.uk./media/S/E/pb.05supportparents391.pdf. Accessed October 2006.

DH (2006b). *Looking for a School Nurse.* London, HMSO.

DH (2007). *Maternity Matters* at http://www.everychildmatters.gov.uk/_files/C5A2FA08979FF29B1711ED9D8F631BF6.pdf

DH, DfES (2003a). *Every Child Matters.* London, The Stationary Office.

DH, DfES (2003b). *Keeping Children Safe.* London, The Stationary Office.

Dunnett, K., White, S., Butterfield, J. and Callowhill, I. (2006). *Health of Looked After Children.* Lyme Regis, Russell House Publishing.

Eisenberg, M. E., Sieving, R. E., Bearinger, L. H., Swain, C. and Resnick, M. D. (2006). Parents' communication with adolescents about sexual behavior: a missed opportunity for prevention? *Journal of Youth and Adolescence,* 35(6): 893–902.

Every Child Matters (2007). 2007 – Under 18 and 16 Statistics. Accessed from http://www.everychildmatters.gov.uk/health/teenagepregnancy/ http://www.everychildmatters.gov.uk/ete/extendedschools/

Giddens, A. (1990). *The Consequences of Modernity.* Cambridge, Polity.

Gillies, V. (2006) Parenting, class and culture: exploring the context of childrearing. *Community Practitioner,* 79(4): 114–117.

Anti-social Behaviour Act. 2003. (Chapter 38). London, HMSO.

Hallam, S., Rogers, L. and Shaw, J. (2006). Improving children's behaviour and attendance through the use of parenting programmes: an examination of practice in five case study local authorities. *British Journal of Special Education,* 33(3): 107–113.

Hamer, M. (2005). *Preventing Breakdown a Manual for Those Working with Families and the Individuals Within Them.* Lyme Regis, Russell House Publishing.

Harrison, C., Parker, P. and Honey, S. (2005). Stepping stones: parenting skills in the community. *Community Practitioner*, 78(2): 58–61.

Hauser (1991). Cited in Taylor, J. Miller, D. (1995). *Nursing Adolescents. Researched and Psychological Perspectives*. Oxford, Blackwell Science.

Hunt, C. and Mountford, A. (2003). *The Parenting Puzzle: How to Get the Best Out of the Family – the Family Links Nurturing Programme*. Oxford, Family Links.

Jones, L. (2006). Developing everyones learning and thinking abilities: a parenting programme. The southern experience – 10 years on! *Child Care in Practice*, 12(2): 141–155.

Juby, H. and Farrington, D. P. (2001). Disentangling the link between disrupted families and delinquency. *British Journal of Criminology*, 41: 22–40.

Kendall, S. and Blookfield, L. (2005). Developing and validating a tool to measure parenting self efficacy. *Journal of Advanced Nursing*, 51(2): 174–181.

Korner, S. (2007). *Information Alert: How Parents and Children Can Function as a Successful Team*. Psychology Online. Accessed from http://www.psychologyinfo.com/treatment/parentsandchildren.html

Kowaleski-Jones, L. and Dunifon, R. (2006). Family structure and community contexts evaluating influences on adolescent outcomes. *Youth Society*, 38: 110.

LeResche, L., Mancl, L., Drangsholt, M., Saunders, K. and Korff, M. (2005). Relationship of pain and symptoms to pubertal development in adolescents. *Pain*, 118(1): 201–209.

Long, A., McCarney, S., Smyth, G., Magorrian, N. and Dillon, A. (2001). The effectiveness of parenting programmes facilitated by health visitors. *Journal of Advanced Nursing*, 34(5): 611–620.

National Healthy Schools Programme (NHSP) (2005). Accessed at http://www.healthyschools.gov.uk/

Parker, S. and Kirk, S. (2006). The parent positive programme: opportunities for health visiting. *Community Practitioner*, 79(1): 10–14.

Pollard, N. (1998). *Why Do They Do That? Understanding Teenagers*. Oxford, Lion Publishing.

RCP (The Royal College of Psychiatrists) (2007). *Surviving Adolescence – A Toolkit for Parents*. www.rcpsych.ac.uk/mentalhealthinformation/childrenandyoungpeople/adolescents

Resnick, M. D., Bearman, P. S., Blum, R. W. *et al*. (1997). Protecting adolescents from harm. Findings from the National Longitudinal Study on adolescent health. *Journal of American Medical Association*, 278(10): 823–832.

Schuster, M. A., Eastman, K. L. and Corona, R. (2006). Talking parents, healthy teens: a worksite-based program for parents to promote adolescent sexual health. *Preventing Chronic Dis*ease, October, 3(4): A126.

Social Exclusion Unit (2004). *Autumn Report – Truancy and School Exclusion Report*. www.socialexclusion.gov.uk. Accessed January 2004.

Social Exclusion Unit (2007). *Reaching Out – An Action Plan on Social Exclusion*. Accessed from: http://www.cabinetoffice.gov.uk/social_exclusion_task_force/publications/reaching_out/reaching_out.aspx

Strange, J. J. (2007). Adolescents, media portrayals of. In Arnett, J. J. (ed.) *Encyclopaedia of Children, Adolescents, and the Media.* Thousand Oaks, CA, Sage.

Strasburger, V. C. (2006a). Risky business: what primary care practitioners need to know about the influence of the media on adolescents. *Primary Care: Clinics in Office Practice*, 33(2): 317–348.

Strasburger, V. C. (2006b). 'Clueless': why do pediatricians underestimate the media's influence on children and adolescents. *Pediatrics*, 117: 1427–1431.

Strasburger, V. C. and Wilson, B. J. (2002). *Children Adolescents and the Media.* Thousand Oaks, CA, Sage.

Teenage Pregnancy Unit (2004). *Teenage Pregnancy: Autumn Strategy Document*. DfES Publications. London, The Stationary Office.

Turner, J. S. and Helms, D. B. (1995). *Lifespan Development*, 5th edition. Florida, Harcourt Brace.

UNICEF (2007). *Report Card 7, Child Poverty in Perspective: An Overview of Child Well-being in Rich Countries.* Accessed from: http://www.unicef.org.uk/publications/pdf/rc7_eng.pdf

Wanless, D. (2003). *Securing Good Health for the Whole Population.* http://www.hm-treasury.gov.uk./consultations_and_legislation/wanless/consult_wanless04_final.cfm

Webster-Stratton, C. and Hammond, M. (1997). Treating children with early onset conduct problems: a comparison of child and parent training interventions. *Journal of Consulting and Clinical Psychology*, 65(1): 93–109.

Willcox, A. and Gleeson, J. (2003). Boys, young men and teenage pregnancies. *Primary Health Care*, 13(8): 27–31.

Woodard E. H. and Gridinia N. (2000). *Media in the Home. The Fifth Annual Survey of Parents and Children.* The Annenburg Public Policy Centre, University of Pennsylvania.

Villani, S. (2001). Impact of media on children and adolescents: A 10-year review of the research. Research update review. *Journal of the American Academy of Child and Adolescent Psychiatry*, 40(4): 392–401.

Young Minds (2005) at http://www.youngminds.org.uk/

Others providing useful information and advice

Burtney, E. and Duffy, M. (eds.) (2004). *Young People and Sexual Health.* Hampshire, Palgrave.

Coleman, J. (2001). *Sex and Your Teenager: A Parent's Guide.* Chichester, John Wiley and Sons.

Coleman, J. and Roker, D. (2001). *Supporting Parents of Teenagers: A Handbook for Professionals.* London, Jessica Kingsley.

Journal of Adolescence. www.apnet.com/adolescence

Parsons, Rob and Parsons, Lloyd. (1999). *What Every Kid Wished Their Parents Knew … and Vice Versa.* London, Hodder Stoughton.

RCN (2002). Getting it right for teenagers in your practice. http://www.rcn.org.uk/__data/assets/pdf_file/0008/78542/001798.pdf

Trust for the study of adolescence. www.tsa.uk.com

Varma, V. (1997). *Troubles of Children and Adolescents.* Bristol, Jessica Kingsley.

Websites

http://guidance.nice.org.uk/topic/behavioural
www.unicef.org.uk
www.dfes.gov.uk/teenagepregnancy
www.dfes.gov.uk
www.everychildmatters.gov.uk
www.teachernet.gov.uk
www.homeoffice.gov.uk
www.cabinetoffice.gov.uk/social_exclusion_task_force/

All of the following handouts and advice boxes can be found as individual pdfs on the website at www.blackwellpublishing.com/thew

Advice box 9.1 General advice for 'good communication'

The following advice is partly guided by Psychology online (2007), Korner (2007) and Royal College of Psychiatrists (2007). First, remind your client that parenting is not an instinct, we have picked up our cues from our own parents. If we as children had a fractious relationship with our parents, we often can have the same with our own offspring. We may need to learn alternative ways to 'parent'. Try to avoid following the 'blame game' where one parent blames another or blames the school. This can lead to little change and can be defensive behaviour. If there are issues with regard to the parents mental health, suggest referral for support.

Help the parent by getting them to talk briefly about their own childhood, and what they would like for their own children, ensure parents/carers have realistic expectations. Dispel the myth that parenting skills classes are just for 'bad' parents – these are a worthwhile learning venture for all parents because it is one of the most difficult jobs of all and learning how to do it well pays enormous dividends. Encourage and support parents and children to function as a successful team. Advise 'active listening' – showing emotions and interest when communicating with young people. Reduce the 'emotional contagion' (often when emotions are running high): listening is affected by overload of emotions, therefore, avoid confrontation and communicate when the emotions have settled down.

Suggest to the parent to consult with the young person – taking on-board the needs and wants as a basis for negotiation, aim for good emotional communication. Examine the young person's feelings and emotions and elicit the objections in a controlled manner. Ensure parents have rules and boundaries in place and ensure consistent parenting from partners/carers/grandparents – it may be better if all the family are involved. Encourage praise and rewards as well as the use of effective and realistic consequences for poor behaviour.

Advice box 9.2 Creating family 'time'

There may be a need to get the whole family to get on-board with healthy eating/exercise and regular routines. With the increasing emergence of 'family life' being eroded by isolating activities, such as watching TV, playing on the computer, listening to music in the bedroom, there is less opportunity for the family to chat. When the emphasis is on cooking, eating and clearing away together, the 'chat' can become naturally more meaningful discussion, as the emphasis is on the activity. This can also reduce family tension, as can a day out of the house together. One of the first tasks may be to suggest that the family go out together, whether that be to the local park for a kick about with a ball, walk the dog, and so on, or away to the seaside. Many families simply follow the 'same old' routine of seeing their own friends, watching TV, doing the housework, and so on; 'family time' is therefore not a happy event!

This family time can involve a grandparent, aunt, and so on especially if the family is a one-parent family. Perhaps getting the children to come up with where they would like to go to may be a starting point.

When to refer on. The following are accepted as being within the limits of normal behaviour and are expected to be managed by the providers of tier 1 services (Department for Education and Employment (DfEE), 2001) within CAMHS:

- Aggressive behaviour
- Unhappiness/misery
- Behaviour problems
- Sleep problems
- Phobias
- Social anxieties
- Bedwetting/soiling.

However, the following should be referred to tier 2 or above as a matter of priority:

- Self-harm
- Depressive behaviour
- Eating phobias or eating disorders such as bulimia or anorexia
- Conduct disorders such as defiance, anti-social and violent behaviour.

Handout 9.1 Roles and rules in parenting – the obvious and not so obvious

Love. This may at times be 'tough' – loving your children does not mean you need to say yes all the time or be their best friend, sometimes it will mean being hard and saying no, or dishing out consequences for poor behaviour. Do not be concerned when your child says they do not love you in a fit of anger – this is very normal!

Care. Meeting your children's 'needs' from food to clothing is an important and vital role – it is important though to realise the difference between a want and a need and that this does not mean you have to meet their every 'want'.

Protection. Keeping a child safe requires teaching them what is and is not safe behaviour and also the ability to be aware of safety as they become independent. This involves strangers, roads, parks, play and also sexual health and regard for their environment.

Be fair. This is the most important concept for children to learn to accept – as a parent if you can help your children see your actions are fair and just, they will more easily accept what is happening to them.

Listen. Active listening requires an ongoing interest in what another person is saying, and asking questions adds richness to the conversation. If anger or disapproval enters into the communication, then emotions are charged and active listening is disrupted. Children and parents have a very good ability to raise each other's anger and emotions and if the communication has been 'hijacked' by the more negative responses, it is time for 'time out' – to end the conversation and resume at a later date when everyone has calmed down. This is proven to be more effective at diverting crises.

Teach. You will need to teach your child the difference between right and wrong, acceptable and unacceptable behaviour, respect for themselves and for other people. Children learn by example and they learn the basics at home before the school years begin – once at school you will guide them into taking responsibility for their behaviour.

Develop their confidence and self-esteem. A child who is criticised, bullied, challenged unfairly or unfairly treated at home or school is more likely to lack confidence and have a poor self-image. This is when they may fall into the 'wrong' set of friends and be unable to say no to risky behaviours. A child who is confident and feels worthy will be more likely to resist peer pressure.

Help your child feel valued. In a large survey of children/young adults in 21 developed countries, the UK came bottom in terms of children feeling loved, nurtured and valued. How do you make a child feel valued? By acting on all the information in this handout and playing a constant role in their lives – whether that be in a static family unit, a reconstituted family unit or a single-parent family unit – it does not matter if all this is provided in equal measure.

Consistency. This is perhaps one of the most challenging facets of being a parent – being consistent in setting boundaries of what is acceptable and what the rules and regulations are for the family – sticking to the boundaries you have set prevents children from playing one parent off against the other or off school staff. If children are met with the same response all around then they actually feel safe and secure even though they may moan a lot about it!

Praise. Positive feedback for behaviour and actions are vital. Rewards for achievements and for overcoming challenges are a sure way of reaping the rewards of a happy and confident child.

Stay involved. Being involved in your child's life is important as long as the child does not see it as an intrusion – be guided by your child. This is a challenge and it does not mean you are wrong to need to know where they are going and who they are going out with no matter how old they are, it is common courtesy. However, it is not uncommon for them to not want you at their school/sporting events as they reach the adolescent years, but asking about it and listening to the excitement or disappointment afterwards is vital and helps you and them feel involved.

Clear, calm and realistic parenting style. Better for your own health and for family harmony – children hate being shouted at. If you can dish out punishments in a calm and reasonable manner it will help to avert the 'screaming abdabs' from either you or them!

Play together. This is possible whether they are 1 or 21 – making time to be together having fun is a good ingredient for success – this might be simple pleasures such as walking, cycling, visiting the park, playing cards or games or more luxurious treats. Being together as a family is the important thing here.

Handout 9.2 Understanding what is going on in your teen

Physical changes

- Puberty – periods, breasts, wet dreams, voice breaking, spots and the rest!
- Rapid growth – can be painful for the child and the parent's pocket!
- Acne and other skin problems
- Tiredness due to increase use of energy – it is normal for them to 'sleep for England'!
- Changes in appearance – leaving a parent wondering where their little one has gone!

Psychological changes

- Friendships may change frequently or become closer
- Relationships are put under pressure
- Disagreements are common
- Tears are a common sight, often for no reason
- Moody and irritable
- Experimentation with food, clothes, friends and other more risky things are very common in the teen years.

Emotional changes

- Stress and distress
- Anxiety
- Depression
- Poor and low self-image
- Lack of confidence.
- Sexual changes
- Awareness of own growing sexuality
- Experimentation
- Promiscuity
- Lack of knowledge and understanding regarding contraception and the legal issues of confidentiality and consent.

Behaviour

- Feelings of loss of control and power
- Power battles
- Testing of boundaries
- School problems and school phobia
- Drugs
- Alcohol
- Smoking
- Substance misuse
- Eating problems
- Trouble – at school or with the law.

Handout 9.3 The art of communicating over difficult issues without falling out with your child

- Consulting with children and young people is a way of gathering information and staying involved. Asking what they would like is not the equivalent of doing what the child asks. Maintaining the difference between talking and doing is extremely important in undertaking the task of consulting with your child.
- Listen actively to your child and master the difficult job of containing your own emotions (keeping them at bay or in check).
- You are now ready to attempt to consult with your child about the issue/topic that may be a problem.
- As we do not know exactly what our child/teen needs at any moment in time – they need to tell us. Remain calm allow their feelings to 'wash' over you without drowning in them!
- Take time to examine their feelings so that you may understand their dilemma.
- Consult with them about what might help without being put-off by the negative responses or the 'out of the question' requests.
- Find out what their objections or complaints are and although this may sound like a crazy idea it is this that will lead to cooperation.
- Discuss together how to remove the obstacles in the road to resolving the problem.
- Once this difficult but 'doable' improvement in communication is achieved, many of the negative behaviours children and teens are engaging in will be likely to drop off. This is because much of this has been carried out to get your attention.

Who to contact if you need support

GP
School Nurse
Health Visitor
Social Services
Youth Workers
Teachers
School Learning Mentor.

Handout 9.3 Continued

Sources of help

Kidscape: www.kidscape.org.uk
Raising Kids: www.raisingkids.co.uk
Frank: www.talktofrank.com
Parentline: www.parentlineplus.org.uk
Royal College of Psychiatrists: www.rcpsych.ac.uk/mentalhealth-information/mentalhealthandgrowingup.aspx
US based web site: www.parentingateenager.net
Child line: www.childline.org.uk
Brook sexual advisory service: www.brook.org.uk
Trust for the Study of Adolescence: www.tsa.uk.com
Young Minds: www.youngminds.org.ukv

10. *Positive Parenting and the Younger Child*

Fiona Wondergem and Dawn Taylor

Introduction

The main aim of the chapter is to inform health and social care professionals on how to empower parents within their role. Specific issues regarding child behavioural issues during the first years of life will be addressed as problems often stem from a lack of parental understanding of so-called normal toddler behaviour, and an inability by parents to manage their own and others' expectations in this stage of parenting.

It is important that parents identify what the problem is and then select particular management techniques appropriate to the issue, the key requirement is therefore related to straightforward, manageable strategies, which can be easily implemented in individual situations and enable a general understanding of the issues relating to toddler development and parenting. Parents need to be encouraged to identify their long-term aim so that a structured plan can be devised in partnership with them. The plan needs to be achievable and realistic with a step-by-step approach.

Topics covered include the management of temper tantrums, sleep, eating problems and toilet training. These key issues are discussed in the following sections. The health professional is encouraged to help parents look for the positive aspects of parenthood and to enjoy the early years and the development of their child. The importance of not presenting parents with confusing and conflicting information is emphasised and helpful routines are discussed.

Sleep disturbances

For many parents, their children's sleep problems are a common cause of considerable stress within the family (Wiggs, 2003). In addition, they are often overlooked by health professionals and effective advice on how to deal with them is not always forthcoming as some health professionals, including doctors, may not feel they have the necessary skills, knowledge and experience to help parents negotiate this challenging period of toddler development.

Intervening through education is a predominant approach in the area of childhood sleep disturbance. This presents its own set of problems: differing prior education levels of the parents and methods of delivering 'education' (e.g. face to face or via a booklet) could affect the efficacy of interventions, and these factors need to be specifically addressed so that the most appropriate form of intervention for particular families can be determined.

Among the most common problems are difficulties in settling children to sleep and repeated waking during the night. Around 40% of children have a sleep problem considered to be significant by their parents (Boyle and Cropley, 2004).

Research has shown that sleep problems are often associated with a range of undesirable factors (Quine, 1992; Wiggs and Stores, 1998) and children with sleep problems are more likely to have behavioural problems than children who sleep well. Other consequences of sleep disruption in children include daytime irritability, hyperactivity, aggression, learning difficulties, reduced attention and concentration. These effects are even more pronounced if present in a child with a learning disability as they may add significantly to the level of developmental delay already experienced and may also be misconstrued as part of the child's condition or a child just being 'difficult' (France and Blampied, 1999).

In many children, sleep problems occur only occasionally, and thankfully for the majority of these children and their parents they are not serious and will improve independently of intervention, given time. But in some instances if the situation does not improve, then sleep problems need to be taken seriously. As well as being distressing, they may interfere with the child's learning and behavioural development, immune function and growth, or may be an indication that there is an underlying health problem, physical or mental (Jan and Freeman, 2004).

There may also be adverse effects on the family such as parental ill-health, reduced affection for the child, marital discord and adverse effect on the parent's work ability (Durand and Mindell, 1990; Carr, 2000; How Ong *et al.*, 2006).

In the main there are three basic types of sleep problem:

- Not sleeping enough (sleeplessness or insomnia)
- Sleeping too much (excessive sleepiness or hypersomnia)

- Episodic disturbances of behaviour related to sleep (parasomnias), for example night terrors.

Settling problems

Settling and waking problems can be caused by a variety of factors and occur in about 20% of 1–2-year olds and 16% of 3-year olds (Mindell, 1999; Boyle and Cropley, 2004). Causes can include incorrect sleep associations, night-time fears, allergy or ill-health.

Waking problems

Waking problems are when sleep is disturbed after the child has gone to bed and fallen asleep and occur in about 20% of 2-year olds and 14% of 3-year olds (Mindell, 1999; Boyle and Cropley, 2004). Some children wake frequently in the night and disturb their parents by crying and calling for attention or by repeatedly coming into their parents' room (Eckerberg, 2004). Some wake only once or twice but cannot be resettled easily (Mindell, 1999).

Disturbances of the sleep–wake cycle

In addition to settling and waking problems, children sometimes show other symptoms of sleep disturbance that interferes with their ability to sleep at the right times (Villo – Sirerol, 2002). These include variable sleep–wake patterns, feeling tired unusually early but waking early (before 5 a.m.), or not going to sleep until unusually late but staying in bed in the morning (Reid *et al.*, 1999).

Excessive daytime sleepiness

Excessive daytime sleepiness can have considerable psychological and social effects on any individual; however, it is rarely seen as a medical problem by parents or professionals, and symptoms may be misinterpreted as laziness, disinterest or lack of motivation. However, sleepiness in children can manifest itself by causing a variety of undesirable behaviours such as irritability, aggression, poor concentration and hyperactivity (Smits *et al.*, 2003). Such problems may be wrongly attributed to causes other than sleeplessness, especially in children with learning difficulties.

Excessive daytime sleepiness may be the result of insufficient sleep or it may be the result of more specific sleep disorders which have an intrinsic, physical origin. One such disorder, obstructive sleep apnoea syndrome, is of particular relevance to children with Down's syndrome and is due to various anatomical characteristics associated with the condition including muscle laxity, enlarged tonsils and adenoids and a smaller upper airway (Lim and McKean, 2003; Montgomery *et al.*, 2004).

In children who are developing normally, sleep-schedule problems result from a mismatch between the individuals' circadian sleep–wake system and the environmental demands regarding the timing and duration of sleep (Jenkins, 2005). There may also be a clash between the child's needs and the parents' desires and expectations of timing and duration of sleep. One way of managing sleep-schedule disorders is chronotherapy. This involves progressively shifting the time of sleep by a set period each day until the desired sleep is achieved and where the sleep periods are then stabilised. The use of sleep aids such as a T-shirt that has been worn by the mother and has her scent on it may also facilitate the development of settled sleep–wake behaviour in young children (France *et al.*, 1996; Wiggs, 2003; Jenkins, 2005).

Nightmares

For most children, dreams are pleasant experiences of everyday events. Whilst nightmares are infrequent, often very real and soon forgotten, for some children they are very disturbing, particularly if frequent or if the child dwells on them for several days, for example, by repetitive acting out of the nightmare with toys, a dread of sleep or struggling to stay awake (Mindell, 1999; Ramchandani *et al.*, 2000). Parents can help by encouraging their child to talk about the dream or draw a picture of it. This will help them to find out the cause of the upset and work out what help or support their child needs (Ramchandani, 2000).

Night terrors

Night terrors are completely different from nightmares or anxiety-related dreams. The first sign is that the child is screaming uncontrollably and seems to be awake, however, despite appearances, the child is asleep.

As many parents find the sight of their distressed child very upsetting, reassurance should be given that the child will not remember the 'monster under the bed' the next day as morning recollection of night terrors is fragmentary at best (Ramchandani *et al.*, 2000; Wiggs, 2003).

In the pre-school child, parents' unwillingness to establish and consistently enforce rules for going to bed, or staying in bed during the night should also be considered, as these actions can lead to irregular sleep patterns and night-time disturbances. In these instances health visitors can be of great assistance to families by recommending techniques to them that have been shown to be effective (Handout 10.1).

Management of sleep disorders

Different sleep problems require different approaches. A sleep problem with a physical cause, for example, obstructive sleep apnoea, will require a very different approach from to say, a settling or waking problem (Blunden, 2004). Therefore it is important to establish:

- The nature and development of the sleep problem.
- Whether the child's sleep environment and activities have any adverse effect on the child's sleep pattern and for this a simple sleep diary kept over a 2-week period which details periods of sleep and wakefulness can be very useful.

Behavioural approaches

More specific and individually designed behavioural and cognitive approaches may be needed for some sleep disorders (Lucas *et al.*, 2003).

In general, a behavioural intervention is one where the principles of learning theory are applied to bring about a change in how a person responds to a particular object or event. A cognitive behavioural intervention is one where treatment approaches use both cognitive (e.g. working with thoughts, attitudes and beliefs) and behavioural methods to change overt (visible) and covert (hidden, e.g. cognition and emotion) behaviours. Interventions that focus on infants, with limited language capacity, tend to be behavioural, whereas with older children, who are more amenable to communication and persuasion, cognitive behavioural interventions can be more practically applied. It is worth noting, however, that even purely behavioural interventions involve a cognitive component when working with parents, since one often has to alter the thoughts, attitudes and beliefs of parents before they are willing and convinced enough to undertake a behavioural treatment programme.

These techniques have been shown to be particularly effective in the management of childhood sleeplessness and aim to change the way parents react and deal with the problem.

Lawton *et al.* (1991) identify four techniques for change: extinction, positive reinforcement, shaping and graded approaches and antecedent conditions and discrimination learning. This approach can also be applied to bring about change in other aspects of child behaviour such as reducing temper tantrums in young children.

Extinction

Extinction involves the removal of any rewarding responses to a child's undesirable behaviour, for example, ignoring a child who cries in the night. Although this can be a very effective approach, it can be upsetting to all concerned and unless used consistently, it can do more harm than good as partial reinforcement of long periods of crying can make the behaviour more resistant to extinction.

A variation on this theme, and one which is often more acceptable to parents, is the controlled ignoring technique or '5-minute checking method' (Jenkins, 2005), where parents settle their child with the minimum amount of interaction and then go back to check their child and carry out the process again every 5 minutes until the child falls asleep on their own. Perseverance and consistency underpin the success of this approach.

Positive reinforcement

Positive reinforcement works on the premise that by rewarding desirable behaviour the behaviour will be repeated and it works best with children who have a verbal age of around 3-years old. Star charts, farmyard charts or anything else that the child finds rewarding can be used. The desired behaviour is made clear to the child so that they know exactly what is required of them in order to achieve the reward.

It is recommended that reinforcement be given for the existence of certain behaviour, rather than its absence, for example, child stays in their own bed rather than not getting into parents' bed. There are of course other reasons why a child should be discouraged from sharing their parents bed, such as reducing the incidence of sudden infant death syndrome or cot death particularly in the under-2 age group (Fleming *et al.*, 2004).

Shaping and graded approaches

Shaping and graded approaches involve teaching the child the desired behaviour in small steps for example gradually moving bedtimes earlier on successive nights for the child who will not settle until late at night (Heussler, 2005). These techniques require careful monitoring so that there is no regression to the earlier problems. They are sometimes much slower than some of the other techniques and so parents may require greater amounts of guidance and support.

Antecedent conditions and discrimination learning

This method involves teaching children to associate sleeping and settling on their own with certain events and conditions. Establishing a good bedtime routine is an example of antecedent learning and if the routine is kept relatively constant and the child knows that they are expected to settle to sleep at the end of the routine, they are more likely to comply. However, it is important that the routine should not be drawn out so that the first part of it becomes disassociated with going to bed and falling asleep.

Behavioural methods to improve parents' handling of bedtime and night-waking problems are very effective (Handout 10.1). Gradually changing children's need for their parents' presence at bedtime or during the night is usually beneficial if used consistently and with conviction (Ramchandani *et al.*, 2000). The techniques described can be used in conjunction with each other in an effective way, for example, for a child who will not settle at night, a bedtime routine can be introduced, 5-minute checking method can be used to teach the child to fall asleep on their own and a star chart can be introduced to reward the desired behaviour.

Above all, it must be remembered that professional advice and support perhaps from a health visitor or, in the occasional severe or complex situation, a psychologist, is very important for any plan of sleep management to be successful.

Toilet training

Toilet training is a universally acquired skill for the normally developing child, yet there is still little or no information about the requisite skills that children learn sequentially, beginning with the signs of readiness and ending with successful completion of toileting (Behrman *et al.*, 2000).

Learning bowel and bladder control is an important part of the socialisation process. In Western culture, a great sense of shame and disgust has been associated with body waste products (Horn *et al.*, 2006) and to function successfully in this culture, one must learn to dispose of body waste products in a place considered proper by society (Sun and Rugolotto, 2004; Potter, 2005). During toilet training, the child, who is just learning about control of the personal environment, finds that some of that control must be given up to please the most important people in his life – his parents (Monsen, 2001). The toddler must learn to conform not only to please those special loved ones' and to preserve self-integrity, but must also persuade himself that this acceptance of the dictates of society is voluntary.

Timing

Most parents eagerly anticipate potty training – if for no other reason than that it signals an end to changing nappies. But few are prepared for how long it can take and although some children get the hang of it within a few days, there are many more who may take several months. Parents and their children have a better chance of success if they know the basics of training and can make the process clear to their toddler (Handout 10.2).

Paediatric literature stresses the importance of a child's readiness before initiating toilet training (Behrman *et al.*, 2000; Schum *et al.*, 2002), including the achievement of motor milestones (such as sitting and walking, understanding and using words for elimination, positive relationships with caregivers and significant others) and the desire to be autonomous and master primitive impulses (Schum *et al.*, 2002; Horn *et al.*, 2006). It is also important that there is not too much pressure for the child to 'perform' before they are ready, likewise, relapses, even after control is achieved, is likely to happen; however, if frequent, potential problems with colonic transit times, bacterial infection and previously undiagnosed anorectal malformations should be ruled out (Benninga *et al.*, 2004; Brandt *et al.*, 2007).

To be able to cooperate in toilet training, the child must possess the necessary physical and cognitive skills and the sphincter muscles must have developed to the stage when the child can control them, for example, staying dry for 2 hours, physical awareness such as appearing uncomfortable in soiled nappies and instructional readiness such as having the ability to indicate a need to urinate (Brazleton *et al.*, 1999; Michel, 1999; Stadtler *et al.*, 1999).

Control of the rectal sphincter develops first and the child must be able to postpone the urge to defecate until reaching the toilet or potty and must be able to signal the need *before* the event. This level of maturation seldom takes place before the age of 18–24 months.

At the start of training, the child has no understanding of the uses of the potty or toilet, but to please his parents the child will sit there for a short time. If bowel movements occur at about the same time every day, one day a bowel movement will occur while sitting on the potty. Although at this stage there is no sense of special achievement, the child will enjoy the praise and approval (Bakker and Wyndaele, 2000). Eventually, the child will connect this approval with the bowel movement in the potty and will be happy that the parent is pleased. Advice to parents on potty training is found in Advice box 10.1.

Bladder training

Generally, the first indication of readiness for bladder training is when the child makes a connection between the puddle on the floor and something he or she did. In the next stage, the child runs to the parent and indicates a need to urinate, but only after it has happened.

Not much benefit is gained from a serious programme of training until the child is sufficiently mature to control the bladder sphincter and reach the desired place. When the child stays dry for about 2 hours at a time during the day, sufficient maturity may be indicated (Hocking, 2005).

Positive training

It is important to make potty training a positive experience for everyone involved. Parents can prepare their child to use the potty in advance by reading books or watching videos about potty training and talking about how exciting it will be when they no longer need nappies. They can also be encouraged to begin using the words that they plan to use for urination and bowel movements in advance so that the child understands what those words mean.

Consistency is the key when introducing the potty, so it is important that ample time is set aside for this process. In the beginning, it is best if parents ensure they have a few consecutive days in which they have very few other commitments, so that they can dedicate themselves fully to the toilet-training process.

Night-time training

Once a child has mastered daytime control, it is time to work on dry nights. Establishing calm evenings at home can be beneficial since this not only helps children to fall asleep easily, but also helps them to stay dry at night (Hjalmas *et al.*, 2004). Drinking fluids should be limited in the hour or so before bedtime and children should be encouraged to use the potty one last time before heading off to bed (Hourihan and Rolles, 1995; Hjalmas *et al.*, 2004).

The mastery of toilet training is an important developmental milestone for children and parents and presents a critical opportunity for anticipatory guidance; parents need guidance in recognising signs of readiness, in helping their child achieve the necessary skills and in preventing or addressing problems when they occur (Redsell and Collier, 2001; Bael *et al.*, 2007; Vermandel *et al.*, 2007).

Tantrums

The toddler years (1–3 years of age) are a time of rapid change and can be among the most exciting and challenging for parents. The most dramatic advances occur in language and interpersonal skills, but progress is evident in all areas as development proceeds along the traditional lines of affective, motor, cognitive and physical growth (Ticehurst and Henry, 1989; Piaget, 1999).

Cognitively, the toddler makes the transition in the second year from sensorimotor to preoperational thought, as defined by Piaget (1999). The transition is characterised by the acquisition of language and the development of pretend play. The young toddler may only know a few words and relies primarily on motor skills to manipulate the environment. In contrast, a 3-year old can speak in sentences and uses these verbal skills to communicate and achieve goals. Physical growth continues more slowly than during infancy, but at a predictable pace. In contrast, fine motor and gross motor skills progress quickly.

Temper tantrums are a frequent occurrence in the developing child. As a child starts to establish his or her independence from parents and caretakers and attempts more complex tasks (Landy and Menna, 2001; Potegal and Davidson, 2003) they are likely to experience episodes of being overwhelmed emotionally to the point of a tantrum.

This behaviour is so common that the stage is commonly referred to as the 'terrible twos', but could just as often referred to as the 'terrific twos' because of the toddler's exciting language development, the exuberance with which he greets the world and a newfound sense of accomplishment. Parents must learn how to manage the fast-paced switching between anxiety and enthusiasm (Handout 10.3).

First and foremost, it is critical to determine that there is no organic cause for the tantrums. A thorough assessment and evaluation for developmental, psychological and physiological explanations for the tantrums is necessary (Potegal and Davidson, 2003; Taylor, 2007). The frequency of the tantrums and the causal factors are critical to determine whether the parents are placing unreasonable expectations on the child. This can be especially true for children who have developmental delays or for toddlers who are especially large for their age (Denham and Couchoud, 1990; Belsky *et al.*, 1996a).

In the majority of children, however, temper tantrums are a normal response to anger and arise from the child's thwarted efforts to exercise mastery and autonomy (Potegal, 2000). Personality also plays a part: with temper tantrums more common among children who are active, determined and energetic by nature and rarely a problem in children who are normally placid and easy-going (Potegal *et al.*, 1998).

It is important to remember that children have different temperaments and parents may need to adjust their expectations and parenting methods to the needs and personality of their child. This does not mean that parents have to give in to all demands, however, it is possible to be flexible in parenting style without compromising either values or beliefs.

Parenting practices that may encourage tantrums include inconsistency, unreasonable expectations, excessive strictness, being overprotective and overindulgence (Needlman *et al.*, 1991). Strategies for managing temper tantrums are in Advice box 10.2. Boredom, fatigue, hunger or illness may also reduce the child's tolerance for frustration, and management mainly consists of teaching the parents to understand the underlying meaning of tantrums and to modify parental behaviours that may perpetuate or accentuate the problem (Levine, 1995; Belsky *et al.*, 1996b).

Eating problems

Eating is a complex behaviour with skills and attitudes that are learned slowly, over time. For the typically developing child, if the relationship around feeding is positive and the food is appropriate, the child will eat and grow, although the amount and range of food may remain limited (How Ong *et al.*, 2006).

The focus in feeding should not be on getting food into the child. Such an emphasis puts pressure on both the feeder and the child, often resulting in disrespectful feeding tactics (force feeding) that pre-empt the child's initiative (Tucker *et al.*, 2006). Such pressure tactics limit the child's possibility for success and instil long-term negative eating attitudes and behaviours (Hutchinson, 1999; Northstone *et al.*, 2001). Instead, the onus should be on the feeding relationship and on the achievable goal of helping the child learn eating skills and positive eating behaviours (Brazelton and Greenspan, 2001).

The principle underlying all interventions is to establish a smooth and congenial feeding relationship that is appropriate for each child's developmental stage, nutritional needs and neuromuscular development. Infants who have not been offered a wide variety of tastes and textures in early life are more likely to be fussy eaters (Harris *et al.*, 1990; Dudek, 2000; Johnson and Harris 2004).

Neophobic response

Toddlers are naturally phobic about new foods (neophobic), but accept most foods with repeated neutral exposure (Wardle *et al.*, 2003). At around 12 months, young toddlers begin to develop this neophobic response to food (Cooke *et al.*, 2003) and become wary of trying new foods. It is thought this may be a survival mechanism to prevent the increasingly mobile toddler from poisoning himself through eating anything and everything (Blissett and Harris, 2002).

At this stage, toddlers may reject a food on sight without tasting it, and may also reject foods that look slightly different from those that they usually eat (a different brand of biscuit or yogurt in a different carton, for instance).

The neophobic response can be stronger in some toddlers than others (Blissett and Harris, 2002), and parents often become very concerned when their toddlers eat only a small range of foods. As toddlers learn by copying, their parents (Farrow and Blissett, 2005), siblings and peers (Birch *et al.*, 1982) most eventually grow out of this phase if they see other people around them eating a wide range of foods (Wardle *et al.*, 2003) (Handout 10.4). Parents must provide the toddler with appropriate food and feeding structure and limit negative behaviours during meals, while at the same time allowing the child to decide how much and whether to eat (Coulthard and Harris, 2003). Such structure and limits are essential if children are to mature in food acceptance and learn the social behaviours associated with eating (Farrow and Blissett, 2005).

The patterns established during the toddler period build an essential framework for eating that persists throughout childhood. Children need the support of regular and reliable meals and snacks, and they need the limits of not being allowed to beg for food handouts or dictate the family menu. With eating, as with other interactions between parent and child, it is disconcerting for children when parents fail to provide them with structure and discipline (Farrow and Blissett, 2005). The general advice for parents on eating problems can be found in Advice box 10.3.

Conclusion

This chapter has focused on positive interaction and addressing the emotional needs of both parents and toddlers. Techniques that enable parents to develop confidence in their own parenting skills, handling stress and frustration and coming to terms with feelings of guilt stemming from their own behaviour and feelings towards their toddler have been demonstrated (Schmidt *et al.*, 2002). It is often a change in parental behaviour that brings about change in the child's behaviour. Parents need encouragement and should be empowered to respond to good behaviour and search for the positive aspects in their child's development.

Behaviour change can only be managed if parents are consistent in their approach; this will help to avoid giving the child conflicting messages. The task for parents is to teach the child what is appropriate behaviour and to reinforce and engender a positive view of themselves through a fair approach to discipline. Praising, encouraging and the giving of unconditional love can build a young child's self-esteem, this promotes core values and promotes effective communication between both parent and child.

References

Bael, A. M., Benninga, H. L., Bachmann, H. *et al.* (2007). Functional urinary and faecal incontinence in neurologically normal children: symptoms of one functional elimination disorder? *British Journal of Urology International*, 99(2): 407–412.

Bakker, E. and Wyndaele, J. J. (2000). Changes in the toilet training of children during the last 60 years: the cause of an increase in lower urinary tract dysfunction? *British Journal of Urology International*, 86(3): 248–252.

Bakker, E., van Gool, J. D., van Sprundel, M., van der Auwera, C. and Wyndaele, J. J. (2002). Results of a questionnaire evaluating the effects of different methods of toilet training on achieving bladder control. *British Journal of Urology International*, 90(4): 456–461.

Behrman, R. E., Kliegman, R. M. and Jensen, H. B. (eds) (2000). *Nelson Textbook of Paediatrics*, 16th edition. Philadelphia, PA, WB Saunders Co.

Belsky, J., Woodworth, S. and Crnic, K. (1996a). Troubled family interaction during toddlerhood. *Development and Psychopathology*, 8: 477–495.

Belsky, J., Woodworth, S. and Crnic, K. (1996b). Trouble in the second year: three questions about family interaction. *Child Development*, 67: 556–578.

Benninga, M. A., Voskuijl, W. P., Akkerhuis, G. W., Taminiau, J. A. and Buller, H. A. (2004) Colonic transit times and behaviour profiles in children with defecation disordes. *Archives of Disease in Childhood*, 89: 13–16.

Birch, L. L., Birch, D. and Martin, D. (1982). Effects of instrumental eating on children's food preferences. *Appetite*, 3: 125–134.

Blissett, J. and Harris, G. (2002). A behavioural intervention in a child with feeding problems. *Journal of Human Nutrition and Dietetics*, 15: 255–260.

Blunden, S. (2004). Are sleep problems under-recognised in general practice? *Archives of Disease in Childhood*, 89(8): 708–712.

Boyle, J. and Cropley, M. (2004). Children's sleep: problems and solutions. *Journal of Family Health Care*, 14(3): 61–63.

Brandt, M., Dougneau, C., Graviss, E. A. and Naik-Mathuria, B. (2007). Validation of the Baylor continence scale in children with anorectal malformation. *Journal of Pediatric Surgery*, 42(6): 1015–1021.

Brazelton, T. B., Christophersen, E. R. and Frauman, A. C. (1999). Instruction, timeliness and medical influences affecting toilet training. *Pediatrics*, 103: 1353–1358.

Brazelton, T. B. and Greenspan, S. (2001). *The Irreducible Needs of Children: What Every Child Must Have to Grow, Learn, and Flourish*. Cambridge, MA, Perseus Publishing.

Carr, A. (ed.) (2000). *What Works with Children and Adolescents? A Critical Review of Psychological Interventions with Children, Adolescents and Their Families*. London, Brunner-Routledge.

Cooke, L., Wardle, J. and Gibson, E. (2003). Relationship between parental report of food neophobia and everyday food consumption in 2–6 year old children. *Appetite*, 41: 205–206.

Coulthard, H. and Harris, G. (2003). Early food refusal: the role of maternal mood. *Journal of Reproductive and Infant Psychology*, 21(4): 335–345.

Denham, S. A. and Couchoud, E. A. (1990). Young preschoolers' understanding of emotions. *Child Study Journal*, 20: 171–189.

Dudek, S. G. (2000). *Nutrition Essentials for Nursing Practice*, 4th edition. Philadelphia, Lippincott Williams, and Wilkins.

Durand, V. M. and Mindell, J. A. (1990). Behavioral treatment of multiple childhood sleep disorders. Effects on child and family. *Behavior Modification*, 14: 37–49.

Eckerberg, B. (2004). Treatment of sleep problems in families with young children: effects of treatment on family well-being. *Acta Paediatrica*, 93(1): 126–134.

Farrow, C. V. and Blissett, J. M. (2005). Is maternal psychology related to obesgenic feeding practices at 1 year? *Obesity Research*, 37(2): 127–134.

Fleming, P. J., Blair, P. S., Sidebotham, P. D. and Hayler, T. (2004). Investigating sudden infant deaths in infancy and childhood and caring for bereaved families; an integrated multi-agency approach. *British Medical Journal*, 328: 331–334.

France, K. G., Henderson, J. M. and Hudson, S. M. (1996). Fact, act and tact: a three stage approach to treating sleep problems of infants and young children. *Child and Adolescent Psychiatric Clinics of North America*, 5: 581–599.

France, K. G. and Blampied, N. M. (1999). Infant sleep disturbance: description of a problem behaviour process. *Sleep Medicine Reviews*, 3: 265–280.

Gaylord, N. (2001). Parenting classes: from birth to 3 years. *Journal of Pediatric Health Care*, 15(4): 179.

Harris, G., Thomas, A. and Booth, D. A. (1990). Development of salt taste in infancy. *Developmental Psychology*, 26(4): 534–538.

Heussler, H. S. (2005). Common causes of sleep disruption and daytime sleepiness: childhood sleep disorders II. *Medical Journal of Australia*, 2 182(9): 484–489.

Hjalmas, K., Arnold, T., Bower, W. *et al*. (2004). Nocturnal enuresis: an international evidence based management strategy. *Journal of Urology*, 171(6 Pt 2): 2545–2561.

Hocking, G. D. (2005). Constipation and toileting issues in children. *Medical Journal of Australia*, 183(7): 391–392.

Horn, I. B., Brenner, R., Rao, M. and Cheng, T. L. (2006). Beliefs about the appropriate age for initiating toilet training: are there racial and socioeconomic differences? *Journal of Pediatrics*, 142(2): 151–152.

Hourihan, J. O. and Rolles, C. J. (1995). Morbidity from excessive intake of high energy fluids – the squash drinking syndrome. *Archives of Disease in Childhood*, 72(2): 141–143.

How Ong, S., Wickramaratne, P., Tang, M. and Weissmann, M. M. (2006). Early childhood sleep and eating problems as predictors of adolescent and adult mood and anxiety disorders. *Journal of Affective Disorders*, 96(1–2): 1–8.

Hutchinson, H. (1999). Feeding problems in young children: report of three cases and review of the literature. *Journal of Human Nutrition and Dietetics*, 12(4): 337–343.

Jan, J. E. and Freeman, R. D. (2004). Melatonin therapy for circadian rhythm sleep disorders in children with multiple disabilities: what have we learned in the past decade? *Developmental Medicine and Child Neurology*, 46: 776–782.

Jenkins, R. (2005). *Introduction to Sleep Problems*, WHO/UK Collaborating Centre Service Guidance. WHO/UK, Geneva, Switzerland.

Johnson, R. and Harris, G. A. (2004). A preliminary study of the predictors of feeding problems in late infancy. *Journal of Reproductive and Infant Psychology*, 22(3): 183–188.

Landy, S. and Menna, R. (2001). Play between aggressive young children and their mothers. *Clinical Child Psychology and Psychiatry*, 6(2): 223–239.

Lawton, C., France, K. G. and Blampied, N. M. (1991). Treatment of infant sleep disturbance by graduated extinction. *Child and Family Behavior Therapy*, 13: 39–56.

Levine, L. J. (1995). Young children's understanding of the causes of anger and sadness. *Child Development*, 66: 697–709.

Lim, J. and McKean, M. (2003). Adenotonsillectomy for obstructive sleep apnoea in children (Protocol for a Cochrane Review) in The Cochrane Library Issue 4, Oxford.

Lucas, P., Liabo, K. and Roberts, H. (2003). *Behavioural Treatment for Sleep Disorders in Children with Downs Syndrome.* London, Childrens Health Research Unit, Institute of Health Sciences, City University

Michel, R. S. (1999). Toilet training. *Pediatrics in Review*, 20(7): 240–245.

Mindell, J. A. (1999). Empirically supported treatments in pediatric psychology: bedtime refusal and night wakings in young children. *Journal of Pediatric Psychology*, 24: 465–481.

Monsen, R. (2001). Giving children control and toilet training. *Journal of Pediatric Nursing*, 16(5): 375.

Montgomery, P., Stores, G. and Wiggs, L. (2004). The relative efficacy of two brief treatments for sleep problems in young learning disabled (mentally retarded) children: a randomised controlled trial. *Archives of Disease in Childhood*, 89: 125–130.

Needlman, R., Stevenson, J. and Zuckerman, B. (1991). Psychosocial correlates of severe temper tantrums. *Journal of Developmental and Behavioral Pediatrics*, 12: 77–83.

Northstone, K., Emmett, P., Nethersole, F. and the ALSPAC Study Team (2001). The effect of age on the introduction to lumpy solids on foods eaten and reported feeding difficulties at 6 and 15 months. *Journal of Human Nutrition and Dietetics*, 14: 43–54.

Piaget, J. (1999). The child's conception of physical causality in the construction of reality in the child, The International Library of Psychology XVIII. London, Routledge.

Potegal, M. (2000). Toddlers' tantrums: flushing and other visible autonomic activity in an anger-crying complex. In Barr, R., Hopkins, B. and Green, J. (eds) *Crying as a Sign, a Symptom, and a Signal: Clinical, Emotional, and Developmental Aspects of Infant and Toddler Crying*. London, MacKeith Press, pp. 121–136.

Potegal, M. and Davidson, R. J. (2003). Temper tantrums in young children: 1 behavioural composition. *Journal of Developmental and Behavioural Pediatrics*, 24(3): 140–147.

Potegal, M., Davidson, R. J., Goldsmith, H. H., Chapman, R. S. and Senulis, J. A. (1998). Tantrums, temperament, and temporal lobes. Paper presented at the *13th Meeting of the International Society for Research on Aggression*, 12–17 July 1998, NJ, Ramapo.

Potter, N. (2005). Differences in child rearing. Cultural contrasts, bringing up children the Honduran way. *Journal of Family Health Care*, 15(1): 26–28.

Quine, L. (1992). Severity of sleep problems in children with severe learning difficulties: description and correlates. *Journal of Community and Applied Social Psychology*, 2: 247–268.

Ramchandani, P., Wiggs, L. and Webb, V. (2000). A systematic review of treatments for settling problems and night waking in young children. *British Medical Journal*, 320(7229): 209–213.

Redsell, S. A. and Collier, J. (2001). Bedwetting, behaviour and self esteem: a review of the literature. *Child Care Health Development*, 27: 149–162.

Reid, M. J., Walter, A. L. and O'Leary, S. G. (1999). Treatment of young children's bedtime refusal and nighttime wakings: a comparison of "standard" and graduated ignoring procedures. *Journal of Abnormal Child Psychology*, 27: 5–16.

Schmidt, L. J., Garratt, A. M. and Fitzpatrick, R. (2002). Child/parent assessed population health outcome measures: a structured review. *Child Care Health and Development*, 28(3): 227–237.

Schum, T. R., Kolb, T. M., McAuliffe, T. L. *et al.* (2002). Sequential acquisition of toilet training skills: a descriptive study of gender and age differences in normal children. *Pediatrics*, 109: e48.

Smits, M. G., van Stel, H. F. and van der Heijden, K. (2003). Melatonin improves health status and sleep in children with idiopathic chronic sleep-onset insomnia: a randomized placebo-controlled trial. *Journal of American Academy of Child and Adolescent Psychiatry*, 42: 1286–1293.

Stadtler, A. C., Gorski, P. A. and Brazelton, T. B. (1999). Toilet training methods, clinical interventions, and recommendations. *American Academy of Pediatrics*, 103(6 Pt 2): 1359–1368.

Sun, M. and Rugolotto, S. (2004). Assisted toilet training in a Western family setting. *Journal of Developmental and Behavioral Pediatrics*, 25(2): 99–101.

Taylor, T. (2007). Managing unwanted behaviour in pre-schoolers. *Community Practitioner*, 80(4): 30–35.

Ticehurst, R. L. and Henry, R. L. (1989). Stage related behavioural problems in the one to 4 year old child: parental expectations in a child development unit referral group compared with a control group. *Australian Paediatric Journal*, 25: 39–42.

Tucker, P., Irwin, J. D., Sangster Bouck, L. M. and Pollett, G. (2006). Previous paediatric obesity recommendations from a community based qualitative investigation. *Obesity Reviews*, 7(3): 251–260.

Vermandel, A., van Kampen, M., van Gorp, C. and Wyndaele, J. J. (2007). How to toilet train healthy children? A review of the literature. *Neurology and Urodynamics*, published online July 2007. Wiley InterScience.

Villo Sirerol, N. (2002). Sleep habits in children. *Annales of Espanoles De Pediatria*, August, 57(2): 127–130.

Wardle, J., Herrera, M. L. and Cooke, L. (2003). Modifying children's food preferences, the effects of exposure and reward on acceptance of an unfamiliar vegetable. *European Journal of Clinical Nutrition*, 57(2): 341–348.

Whelan, E. and Cooper, P. J. (2000). The association between childhood feeding problems and maternal eating disorder: a community study. *Psychological Medicine*, 30: 69–77, Cambridge, Cambridge University Press.

Wiggs, L. and Stores, G. (1998). Behavioural treatment for sleep problems in children with severe learning disabilities and challenging daytime behaviour: effect on sleep patterns of mother and child. *Journal of Sleep Research*, 7: 119–126.

Wiggs, S. (2003). Paediatric sleep disorders: the need for multidisciplinary sleep clinics. *International Journal of Pediatric Otorhinolaryngology*, 67(Suppl 1), pp. 185–190.

All of the following handouts and advice boxes can be found as individual pdfs on the website at www.blackwellpublishing.com/thew

Advice box 10.1 'Potty training'

Suggestions for bowel training include:

- A potty in which a child can comfortably sit with the feet on the floor is preferable as most small children are afraid of a flush toilet.
- The child should only be left to sit for short periods on the potty for only a short time.
- Parents should not hover anxiously over the child. If a bowel movement occurs, approval is in order; if not, then no comment is necessary.
- The potty should be emptied unobtrusively after the child has resumed playing. If it is immediately thrown away, the child may be confused and not so eager to please the next time.

Lapses are inevitable even after control has been achieved. This can be due to the fact that the child is totally absorbed in play or may be due to a temporary episode of loose stool. Parents should be reassured that as long as the lapses are occasional, they should be ignored (Bakker *et al.*, 2002). However, if the lapses are frequent and persistent, or the child is complaining of recurrent abdominal pain the cause should be sought.

Knowing when to start. It is important to follow the child's lead – when he is ready to use a potty he will let his parents know. Other indications that a toddler may be ready to start potty training are

- S/he has regular, soft, formed bowel movements, for example, after breakfast.
- S/he stays dry for a couple of hours each day.
- S/he takes an interest when a parent or older siblings go to the toilet.
- S/he can demonstrate when a bowel movement is taking place.
- S/he lets the parent know that s/he wants to be changed when her/his nappy is soiled.

Advice box 10.2 Managing temper tantrums

Temper tantrums are best handled by ignoring the outburst, offering nurturance to the child after the tantrum has subsided and helping the child learn to express negative feelings in more acceptable ways (Handout 10.3). With some forward thinking, it is possible to help parents to cut down on tantrums or make then less overwhelming by:

- Setting a good example and keeping calm – talking quietly to a child and holding them close can sometimes help.

- Giving plenty of praise for good behaviour.
- Avoiding trouble spots – such as the supermarket.
- Looking for signs of irritation and diverting a toddler's attention elsewhere.
- Offering control and choices – for example, asking a child what clothes they want to wear or what they want for lunch.
- Ignoring the behaviour – sometimes, walking away and pretending to take no notice of a tantrum can cool things down.

There are also many excellent parenting courses being run throughout the country at the present time and access to these can be found through local newspapers, community care services, child guidance clinics, and so on. These courses are an invaluable source of help and support, especially to young parents who live far from the extended family and do not have the advice or the support of their own parents around the corner (Gaylord, 2001).

Advice box 10.3 Advising parents on feeding problems

Establish the parents' own personal feelings about food, perhaps they are a dieter or have a weight problem, if a child tunes into parental anxieties it may be that mealtimes become an ideal time to get attention (Whelan and Cooper, 2000). Toddlers may also be reluctant to eat well if they are:

- Tired
- Distracted by toys, games, TV, a new environment
- Anxious, sad, lonely or insecure
- Not hungry because they have already had enough either at that meal or from eating or drinking before it
- Not hungry because they have drunk too much fluid as milk, juices or squashes or have been grazing too frequently on high-energy snack foods
- Feeling unwell as appetite is often reduced when a child has a temperature or is teething
- Constipated
- Anaemic.

Other influencing factors include factors such as a lack of routine to mealtimes, negative experience around mealtimes or medical problems such as gastro-oesophageal reflux. Most feeding problems do not just develop on their own but develop as a result of an interaction of different factors, for example, a child might be reluctant to try new foods; parents then become anxious and begin to try and control their child's intake.

Advice box 10.3 Continued

Suggest lessening the amount of attention the toddler gets when they refuse to eat – to a 2-year old even the attention of a cross parent is better than no attention at all!

It is important to reassure anxious parents that faddy eating will usually resolve in time by explaining to parents why the food refusal is happening and suggesting changes to the way they manage meal times (Handout 10.4). However, a small minority of toddlers persist in eating very little and this may affect their growth and development. If no medical cause for the problem can be identified, it is likely that the toddler is strongly neophobic about food, and has an extreme sensory sensitivity (Cooke *et al.*, 2003). Under these circumstances, it may be appropriate to refer the child to a clinical child psychologist or a specialist feeding team if available.

As it is entirely normal for toddlers to refuse to eat or even taste new foods, they will learn to eat and enjoy new foods by copying adult behaviour; therefore, eating as a family as often as possible should be encouraged. It is extremely rare for a child to actually starve himself and the majority of children will generally eat enough to keep them going. Just as anxiety may cause problems with toilet training, it can also create difficulties with eating. So it is important for parents to take a step back and think about how much of a problem there really is. Unless a child is clearly not gaining weight as he should or is obviously unwell, parents should try not to worry and treat the reluctance to eat as a normal and transient phase.

Handout 10.1 Behaviour management for sleep disturbance

Do's and don'ts for effective sleep management

Do check your child is not unwell, hungry, thirsty or wet.

Do get your infant into a routine which is acceptable for both you and your partner.

Do be firm and consistent.

Don't try to settle your child by getting into bed or sitting on his bed.

Don't draw out bedtime routines – a child who will not sleep after two stories is not going to sleep after five.

For older toddlers

Do cut out late afternoon naps.

Do provide a nightlight if your child is scared in the dark or leave a landing light on

Do consider trying the controlled ignoring technique or 5-minute checking method. This is where parents settle their child with the minimum amount of fuss and then go back to check their child and carry out the process again every 5 minutes until the child falls asleep on their own. Do consult your health visitor if the problem is persistent.

Handout 10.2 Behaviour management for toilet training

Do's and don'ts for effective toilet training

Do start potty training when your child becomes aware of having a wet or dirty nappy.

Do not start potty training too early.

Do leave the potty around so that the child can see it and knows what it is used for.

Do take your child's nappy off and suggest they use the potty if your child regularly opens his/her bowels at the same time each day.

Do try the same approach as soon as your child knows that he/she needs a wee.

Do offer praise when your child is successful.

Don't be too critical of accidents – they will happen and in the early days will be frequent.

Don't cut back on fluids during the day.

Do remember when your child is dry consistently over several weeks to try and leave their nappy off at night.

Do protect the bed mattress in case of accidents at night.

Do contact your health visitor or GP if your child is experiencing problems with daytime wetness when they are approaching school age.

Handout 10.3 Behaviour management for tantrums

Do's and don'ts for effective management of tantrums

Do remember that tantrums are more likely to occur if a child is tired or hungry.

Do avoid tantrum hotspots such as the supermarket if your child is prone to tantrums.

Do try to distract your child before a tantrum begins.

Do remember to lead by example.

Don't lose your temper.

Do try to understand your child's feeling of anger and frustration.

Do offer choices/alternatives and try not to always say no.

Do encourage your child to let their feelings out in other ways.

Do take time out by placing your child in a safe place for a short time.

Do talk to your child.

Do show your child how much you love him/her as extra love maybe what is needed at this time.

Do contact your health visitor or GP if you are seriously worried about your child's behaviour.

Handout 10.4 Behaviour management for eating problems

Do's and don'ts for mealtimes

Do have regular/set mealtimes.

Do try to eat as a family.

Do give your child a place at the table – away from distractions such as the TV.

Don't overface your child by piling food onto their plate.

Do introduce your child to different food tastes.

Don't allow your child to fill up on drinks before mealtimes.

Don't offer sweet courses before savoury.

Don't make mealtimes a war zone.

Even if a food has been refused previously – do offer again.

Don't let your own relationship with food influence your child's eating patterns.

Do talk to your health visitor or GP if you are worried about your child's eating habits.

Index